Lymphatic Drainage System

Understanding Lymphatic Drainage Massage

(Proven Techniques and at-home Strategies for Improving Your Lymphatic Function)

Carlos Robinson

Published By **Bella Frost**

Carlos Robinson

Lymphatic Drainage System: Understanding Lymphatic Drainage Massage (Proven Techniques and at-home Strategies for Improving Your Lymphatic Function)

ISBN   978-1-998038-53-4

No part of this guidebook shall be reproduced in any form without permission in writing from the publisher except in the case of brief quotations embodied in critical articles or reviews.

Legal & Disclaimer

The information contained in this book is not designed to replace or take the place of any form of medicine or professional medical advice. The information in this book has been provided for educational & entertainment purposes only.

The information contained in this book has been compiled from sources deemed reliable, and it is accurate to the best of the Author's knowledge; however, the Author cannot guarantee its accuracy and validity and cannot be held liable for any errors or omissions. Changes are periodically made to this book. You must consult your doctor or get professional medical advice before using any of the suggested remedies, techniques, or information in this book.

Table Of Contents

Chapter 1: The Lymphatic System, And The Way It Operates

The content of this chapter has been designed with utmost care for people who are not medical professionals, and focuses on the fundamentals in the lymphatic systems. There are an abundance of literature that explains the lymphatic system in extensive in depth, it's not my intention to mislead the people who do not have a medical background through a plethora of details about the anatomy and physiology lymphatic system. However, I believe it is important to make you conscious of the importance this system is for the very foundation of our existence, and the reason it is so important to function at a high level of percent throughout the day.

The majority of people recognize the lymphatic system than the immune system. They are, however, exactly the same. The lymphatic system crucial to the body, and crucial to our existence. It's accountable for many aspects:

1. Our body is protected from the invasion of foreign objects (splinters and so on.)

2. It stops germs and bacteria from getting into our body through creating an army inside our bodies (this is referred to as immune).

3. It enlists the troops to battle bacteria and germs which enter the defence of our first line.

4. It cleanses our body of waste products that the waste that our body"s different systems that produce it daily. daily day basis.

Fighting Bacteria

Bacteria or germs get into our body through a variety of ways. In the event of an infection, the body"s immune cells recognize the organisms as hostile and release specially-formulated cells to combat them. when the infection is not serious it will be in a position to create enough cells to fight the invader and eliminate the bacteria. There will be a number of casualties from both the invading bacteria and body"s defense cells. They are then removed and disposed of in drainpipes referred to as lymphatic vessels. They are filled with a fluid called lymph. This is the lymph that carries the lymph nodes (glands) which are cleansed and filtering, and later empty into the primary rubbish disposal inside the chest cavity. Then, they're cleared from the body by the usual pathways.

The Waste Disposal System

There are many organs and system that are operating in tandem to make us able to function. For instance the cardiovascular system, which includes the heart as well as blood (veins and arteries). The heart pumping new blood through the body through arteries. It later collects old blood through veins returning it into the heart for it to begin the entire process over. This is a system that never stops. that is never stopped (thankfully). It is true that, similar to the cardio-vascular system all of the other organ systems in our body generate waste/toxins just like cars produce carbon monoxide (exhaust fumes) as a waste product. Just as exhaust fumes can be deadly for us, so too do the waste/toxins when they are left in the body.

The body normally manages to get rid of the waste/toxins through collection points within the body that are known as glands or nodes. They are known as reservoirs, cleaning out waste and also contain fighting cells that fight invaders of bacteria when they enter the body. I"m certain you've had the surgeon say, "You have an infection due to your glands being up," whilst feeling either the neck side or beneath your armpits? investigation revealed nine out of ten locations within the body that are in which nodes gather are located (see the plate 1). The locations are at either end of the neck; within every armpit, following the the rib cage within the stomach area (this region is quite large and can be categorized as a pair of sites) within each groin, and in the rear of every knee. Each lymphatic gland is used as a filter for waste as well as toxins. When they are full, they then empty to the main organs of waste elimination in the chest cavity to be eliminated by the normal channels.

The smaller lymph nodes (nodules) can be found all over the body, particularly in the throat, intestines as well as the urinary tract (water is a good example). They are thought to be placed strategically to protect the body from diseases that attack the passageways' lining, which connect to the outside part of our body (see Plate 2.). The majority of nodules are tiny and are solitary. There are some which are located in huge collections, like the Tonsils comprise an accumulation of lymph nodules. They're situated strategically below the chin or on to either side of neck, and produce combat cells (lymphocytes) that serve as the first defense against invaders bacteria. The size of nodules varies Some are as tiny as pinheads, while some are as large as one-third the dimension that of an almond.

Lymph Oedema The swelling and inflammation of the tissues of limbs

Because this is an extremely debilitating condition, I decided that I ought to dedicate some time to this issue and explain the reason why it occurs. In the event of increased tension within the lymph system, the tubular walls begin to become clogged and the fluid flows to adjacent tissues. The sluggish fluid eventually causes scarring as well as other modifications in the tissues. Over time, lymphatic vessels are now rigid, impermobile; and the lymph congeals within the vessels that are inflamed and whose pores are similarly blocked due to scar tissues. As a result of these changes, lymphoedema can occur, and in the event of the possibility of infection or injury the condition can become more severe. This is even more complex. The loss of protein within tissues can have devastating effects because the body facing mechanical malfunction of its lymphatic system attempts to counter the issue. The body"s cells try their best to fight these proteins, and as a result, the body"s internal pressure changes, and creates an oedema (swelling) and this could be described as the cabin pressure on an airplane, which causes your ankles to swell. For healthy adults, 1-3 liters of lymph flow into circulatory system daily and is characterized by the protein content of around 4.5%, a significant quantity. When there is an illness-related condition the flow of lymph can be greater than the normal amount by 20 times!

For a summary:

The lymphatic system serves two major functions: combating inflammation through the immune system as well as getting rid of all the body"s debris.

The lymphatic system is devoid of a pump, and relies instead on muscles for the movement of lymph throughout the body.

There are nine or ten major lymph-collecting chambers referred to as (gland) node locations.

If the system is too sagged the muscles get tired; vessels expand, preventing the closing the valves, and the lymph circulation ceases inducing swelling of joints (lymph swelling or oedema).

The scarring caused by stagnant lymph causes inside the tissues. the lymph congeals and continues shutting off the vessels by forming the scar tissues.

The pressure of backpressure builds which causes lymph oedema to increase. We now understand how the lymphatic system can result in severe harm to the body when it's damaged in any way. suggesting the necessity of the right treatment that does not just reverse the negative effects of the degrading lymphatic system, but one which will repair the lymphatic system, ensuring that it is fully functioning.

The distinction in lymphatic drainage and Sepia Technique

In a short time, I'd like to emphasize the distinction between these

two.

Manual Lymphatic Drainage (MLD)is an advanced form of therapy where the practitioner employs various specialized and gentle pumping techniques to alter the direction of the skin's movement towards the direction of lymphatic flow. The lymphatic vessels are stimulated that transport essential nutrients to defenses of the body. It also assists in removing waste materials."

The MLD is a compression-bandaging technique that helps to reduce the risk of infection.

This procedure involves putting bands of tightness around legs to function as compressors, allowing them to compress the stagnant interstitial fluid in the limb. The goal is to push them through the nodes toward the emptying chambers. (See sketch B, next page) Patients of mine who have had this experience say it's an extremely unpleasant feeling. Furthermore, I am concerned that applying bandsags that compress on this kind of problem, that has resulted in poor blood flow through both veins as well as the blood vessels (circulatory impairment) could result in blood bleeding (a semi solid mass created in liquids like lymph or blood through the process of coagulation) and could cause embolism (an obstruction to a blood vessel due to a moving the clot which could cause death) Kasner and Tindall 1985.

Sketch A

While I do agree in the irrefutable benefits that unblocking lymphatic flow offers, I am not convinced that merely moving your skin to the direction of flow will have any long-lasting result. In the event that lymphatic drainage manual originated from places away from your body, like feet and hands, solely the method of drainage will simply move lymph to the nearest nodes, and as these are likely to be blocked (or perhaps partially blocked) it will result in reverse flow (sketch A) and hence the necessity to use compress bandsaging (sketch B) It's similar to moving water towards the blocked drain. It's a waste of time and effort procedure to clear a drain (pushing the skin toward the nodes, as is the MLD) or employing the plunger (compression bandaging) when the major drainage channels (the glands or node locations) are blocked.

Sketch B

The common sense dictates we first need to clear of the main drains. after that, once this is accomplished, the build-up of debris will move through the drainage system. It will then eventually pass into the drains, where they can be cleared.

Chapter 2: What Triggers The Lymphatic System In The Body To Get Blockage?

Although it is a bit intricate is crucial because it can help you discover the reasons that caused your lymphatic system to get blocked and creating the impression that you are, so that once you're cleared, you are able to avoid repeating the experience it. As always, I've tried to make it straightforward, but you'll see that some times it's challenging.

The man who came up with the idea came from Hans Selye (1956), an early researcher in the field of stress, who suggested that there are two types of anxiety: Eustress and distress. Simply put, eustress is vital for our bodies to function in every daily existence. It's the reason we have our enthusiasm for living as well as our passion and excitement; and the "buzz" or buzz" we experience when doing something a little risque. It is more commonly known as ,,the adrenalin rush," however it can be described as exactly that. Eustress (or the good kind of stress) lets us experiment in our lives and provides an "lift" we need to satisfy our craving to gain fulfilment and excitement (why do people want to climb the most dangerous side of the mountain?). In every day life we meet challenges, known as stressors. When the stressor has been dealt with a chemical is released within the body causing feelings of euphoria to occur and produces the ,,feel-good" aspect that the body. When the strain is excessive and we feel "out out of our element" or unable to cope with the situation or challenge, negative feelings such as anxiety, depression, hopelessness, insecurity etc., overwhelm us and cause an overload of another chemical to be released (ACTH). This chemical slows down and stops some of our systems from working causing what we know tobe ,,distress". If we seek assistance to manage the stress and reduce stress, it will be less and feelings of depression are quickly gone, along with the release of another chemical in the body, which restores all the body"s functions to their normal. If the problem persists over a prolonged period with no intervention or even over a prolonged period, it could cause harm to the body. A persistent attack by the stressor is able to continue to release ACTH which triggers the process of shutting down other system within our body. which include the digestive system, tissues repair and most particularly the lymphatic (immune) system.

There are two methods the body reacts to stress. Both of which are activated through hormones produced from (the adrenal) glands that are located above the kidney. Each has an individual hormone. A hormone can increase the heart rate that in turn raises the blood pressure, and also stops digestion. The second hormone controls the heart rate and restores blood pressure to normal, and allows for digestion. While Selye discovered that stress can trigger an emotional response in the body, He did not recognize stress could be caused by emotions or psychological circumstances that trigger the hormone in a normal manner, but the energy that is produced isn't employed. In the event that the stress is prolonged (chronic) and includes a mental stressors, such as those the reason of emotional trauma, for instance, death or trauma,

Depression or financial issues or financial problems, and then the adverse effects of these stress-related situations as well as the shutting down of the non-essential system. Lymphatic (immune) system happens to be among the systems which shuts down in the "stressful phase," as a protection until after the emergency. Normally this is an excellent survival system however, as long as the ,,emergency" is present it will be inactive, making the lymphatic system useless as it is unable to eliminate the body of toxins or protect itself from infection!

Stress Related Illness

The negative effects of stress on the human body have been very well-documented. We all have heard that stress can trigger: an increased blood pressure, atherosclerosis, a hardening or narrowing of the arteries; coronary heart disease which leads in heart attack (Myocardial Infarction) as well as asthma, migraine gastric ulcers and eczema just to name some. In fact, even events that last only a few minutes like a brief marriage break-up may result in a suppression of the immune system, also known as immune suppression (Willis and colleagues 1987).

(Caldwell and colleagues, (Caldwell and colleagues, 2003) acknowledged the dangers of chronic immunosuppression since it renders your body prone to illness and infections. One of the best examples they could provide is AIDS that makes those suffering from it susceptible to many diseases.

In addition, they did a study of the effect of stress while conducting important tests and found definitively that stress caused a substantial decrease in the lymphatic (immune) system. Holmes as well as Rahe (1967) claimed that daily adjustments can cause diverse levels of stress as well as the likelihood of developing illnesses. If we consider marriage to be a normal life event to adapt our lives accordingly the marriage, which was assigned an amount of points equal to 50. Check out the table on the next page. The study also looked at comparisons performed for life-related events with each of the events being either less or more than 50. The researchers found a significant link between higher scores with heart attacks. If you score 150 or greater increased risk of a stress-related breakdown in health by 30%, while the presence of a higher number than 300 raised the risk to 50%. Look over the Holmes and Rahe social adjustment table to check if any of these circumstances are applicable to you and then calculate the score.

Thus, various theorists are studying stress and its extremely dangerous negative impact on the human body. All of them, regardless, have proven conclusively that the type A personality is more susceptible to heart attack, coronary heart disease as well as other heart diseases. Thus, it's reasonable to conclude that those with personality types A definitely require a change in their lifestyle approach if they hope to live longer! Although I've examined the impact of stress on our bodies and people who have Type A personalities however, I am left with the question how does stress bring to people who have the personality type B?" Swindle (1990) carried out research into eight common areas of life stressors. These were: illness and other medical problems, home and local environment (items such as traffic and safety), family finance, relationship with partner, children, extended family, work, and relationships outside the family. He found that there were many sources of stress in life, but all stress without exception would affect physical and psychological health. In addition he highlighted that stress at work will affect performance whatever your job! Furthermore, Matthews and Haynes (1986) found, ,,people vulnerable to illness are those individuals who repress high levels of hostility rather than express it. These are mainly type B personalities." In addition, Caldwell and

Caldwell (2003) say, "They are aware that personalities and gender play a major role in responses in response to stressful situations." De Longis (1982) found that the most stressful thing was minor stressors that we encounter that we encounter in our daily routines, like misplacing keys, being late for a bus, filling out numerous forms etc. which led to later illnesses instead of life-changing circumstances.

Based on Health and Safety Executive statistics that more than 13 million work days are lost annually in the UK by stress. It is thought to cause 70 percent of visits to a doctor and 85percent of serious illness. In addition, they estimate that the expense to employers amounts to PS700 Million annually, while the costs of social stress estimated to be PS7 billion annually! The number is increasing every year!

Not only can stress cause enormous damage on our bodies, but it also affects our entire society which is why it's important to think about ways to relax ourselves.

Physical Effects of Stress

The Occupational Stress Working Party (Loughborough University 2002) declares that the consequences that stress has on the body can be:

The heartbeat is increased to push the blood more quickly around our bodies.

The blood flow is concentrated to the larger muscles, and it is less directed to our extremities (we are literally able to feel cold feet when being scared)

We breathe fast and slowly, inhaling more oxygen.

The liver releases stored sugar in the blood.

The pupils expand to allow more light in.

Every sense is heightened

Muscles tense

The blood flow to the digestive organs are constrained

There is a desire to flush the bladder, the stomach, and bowels (less pounds to carry around if you are trying to run for your entire life)

It is a feeling of tightness, tension and nervous

It is sometimes difficult to concentrate.

In Alan Chapman"s site Businessballs.com (1995from 1995 to 2005) it was stated that stress at the workplace decreases productivity, raises management pressures and can cause illness across a variety of ways. There are evidences that stress from work can affect the brain's ability to perform which includes functions related to working performance as well as memory, concentration, and learning. Stress is confirmed to cause sufferers sick; research is growing about the variety of illnesses as well as diseases that are that are caused by stress.

Stress has been proven as a contributor to heart diseases that causes hypertension, and lowers immunity; Stress is also linked to a stroke, irritable bowel syndrome as well as diabetes, ulcers muscles and joint discomfort, miscarriages, allergy, alopecia and early tooth loss." According to Chapman"s website, you can see that the person"s levels of stress tolerance as time passes and how certain individuals are more susceptible to stress than other. The result will be a negative impact upon the body's immune system that can reduce resilience to stress.

Stress can have a variety of physical effects, with the energy levels are low being just one of them. Consequently, the moment a person feels depleted of energy or feels that they can"t perform exercises, then the excessive levels of glucose are likely to persist in their body, in the event that the stress persists (chronic) and the continuous activation of energy can overwhelm the body"s ability to handle the stress and make us more vulnerable to illness and infection (immunosuppression). The system that is that is the most urgently needed by our body, that of the immune system, is the one which has been eliminated! Now we can observe a pattern forming. Stress is a major factor in stress. The lesser energy we've got as well as the less immunity, and which makes us more vulnerable in a vicious cycle without a clear path to escape; up at least until today. Sepia Technique Sepia Technique has been developed to remove the blockages within the lymph nodes. It allows the lymphatic system to function normally, fight illnesses and diseases that invade the body and allow for mobilization of glucose as well as free fatty acids. This results in recovering the energy. The renewed energy brings the desire to "do" more. The result is an overall improvement on the person"s overall health.

The Fight or Flight Mechanism- how your muscles influence the lymphatic system

When danger is recognized, muscles instantly become tense and ready for actions. The brain is alerted of danger, and hormones trigger muscles to take the correct action which is to escape the threat! Additionally, the body stimulates its nervous system. The result is an increase in the blood flow to the muscles as well as less blood flow of blood flow to the intestines, skin and kidneys. The breathing becomes more intense as well as the heart's and pulse rate increase and this increases blood pressure. It sends signals to the brain that there is an increase in energy requirements thus sugars and fats are released into bloodstreams which is converted into energy and utilized by muscles. In tension all time they are in danger. Take a moment to think about to consider what might happen to your body if the consequences of stress were long-lasting or lasted for a long time? That is, in the event that the environment you're experiencing is a simulation of this "fight or fight" system frequently?

Studies conducted of Madders (1987) showed that the negative effects of stress may occur even if you aren't in risk. Simple everyday events like getting late to appointments or getting caught in traffic may cause stress. It is currently recognized that, continuous emotional state can cause a significant impact on your body, often causing organ damage, leading to the development of infections." Furthermore, that ,,prolonged stress disorders will have a profound effect on the immune system".

What can you tell if when you're overly stressed?

One of the biggest negative consequences of stress is not knowing the signs that we're stressed. How do we know the signs of stress? In addition to the obvious symptoms like palpitations, chest pains and higher blood pressure it is that we don"t. However, other people are able to tell when they feel stressed, and notice changes in our behavior habits. It could be due to emotional physical, mental, or a mix of all three. When a stressed individual confronted about it, they usually ignore the issue but also make excuses to justify their behavior. They'll claim that they're in good health and do not require relaxing. The feeling of exhaustion is accepted as a normal part of life, However, this makes it harder to differentiate between the necessary and those that aren't essential. It is possible that they engage with no results, as is commonly observed in tired mothers as well as employees who are many more responsibilities and in whom "martyr syndrome" is readily recognized by other people. There are other signs of stress, such as bad temper anger, occasional grumbling, long time spent working but not as much focus on minor issues and letting major issues go unnoticed, poor sleeping, drinking and smoking rise, food is not eaten or they are annoyed at the smallest aspect. Health breaks down.

Madders" identifies muscle tension as the first signs of stress. The Corporate Health and Fitness magazine (Feb 1993) stated, ,,unchecked physical stress manifests in tight muscles, increased blood pressure, headaches, aches and pains and over a period of time, illness." In the same issue, they stated that in Britain the average of 37 million working days is taken away each year due to illness caused by stress with a price of PS3,000,000! This number has risen dramatically in the years since. The year 1984 was the year Cary Cooper published an article in the journal Personal Management" which stated that stress from work can manifest itself as physical emotional, as well as what Cooper calls mental behavioural signs (see diagram on the next two pages).

Physical Symptoms

A feeling of apprehension that your heart is beating vigorously, infrequently or fast. within the chest

Insomnia and abdominal distension caused by winds

Diarrhoea, abdominal pain, and colic.

Sometimes, you'll pass urine

Lack of sexual desire or impotence (sexual sexual drive) Modification of menstrual cycle in women. Tingling feelings in the arms or legs

Tension in muscles and tension in the neck, or lower back

Chronic headaches that are often recurring, beginning at the neck, and then moving forward to the head

Migraines

The skin can be irritated

There is a lump that has formed in your throat

Trouble focusing and double vision the eyes

Emotional Symptoms

Rapid and extreme swings in mood

Unreasonably worrying over things that really do not have any significance

Chapter 3: What's Your Personality Type?

In my previous chapter, I briefed you on the various varieties of personalities. In this chapter, I will explain how my studies have shown that individuals with certain kinds of personality tend to have the lymphatic system in their body restricted. (Although anyone can be affected when they display even the smallest indications and symptoms) The experts say that there are two different types of personalities including Typ A, or Type B. While I don't doubt this however, it appears that there's a large portion of people who do not fall into either of those classifications. So I've created the continuum below that shows I have come up with what I consider to be a more accurate classification.

Type A, Type B+A Type B+A-Type B type A people tend to be more susceptible to heart attacks. They're party-goers and often burn the candles in both directions. They enjoy life to the max but they don't take time to recharge and their bodies tend to "burn out" fast; or the body is depleted. body"s organs.

On the other side of the spectrum are those who have the type B personality. They are the ones who tend to take care of the people around them. They are adamant about harmony in the social group and try to achieve this. They work for their fellow humans and tend to be submissive quiet kinds.

People who are Type A+B tend to have most of the characteristics of type A traits but have some types B characteristics. Type B+A is a group of people that exhibit mostly types B personality traits but also have characteristics of a type A. To make things easy, I've explained Type A and B personality types only. This will enable readers to determine about where you fall in the spectrum. For the purpose of this guide, the main one you must determine if you a type B BA or an AB?

Type A Personality

Since the beginning of time, scientists have been investigating Type A behavior pattern, known as TABP which puts certain people at risk for coronary heart condition. The pattern is characterized by characteristics like impatience, aggression as well as a sense stress and the drive to gain recognition and progress. The people who display these traits are hyper-aware of time. They move, eat and do the majority of activities quickly.

These are typically workaholics and extremely driven people who, which in turn, push others to the limit. Tests that have been conducted on the basis of interviews with TABP participants also show that individuals with type A are more likely to display physical signs; i.e., facial tension fast speech and prolepsis (interruption of another's" speech) as well as finger drumming teeth and tongue clicking and audible forced exhalation of air.

Type B Personality

Psychologists have researched people"s behaviors for years. When they were children young, teen, or an adult individuals will be taught (conditioned) to behave (behave) in in a manner that is acceptable not only to others as well as to the individual who is teaching them. In addition, they say that behaviour which is reinforced can be repeated, whereas those who are not conditioned can be eliminated.

Skinner (1957)refers the concept of reinforcement in the sense that, "anything which increases chances that the action which preceded it to occur in the future." Also that it strengthens a reaction and punishment refers to anything that decreases the chance the response is likely to occur. Skinner also stated that there are two types of reinforcement as well as two types of punishment. Positive reinforcement consisted of anything that was enjoyable and increased the likelihood of an action. Like warm food, comfort, music, etc. Negative reinforcements were the removal or escape from things that were unpleasant, which could increase the chance of an action occurring. Like, for example, getting away from electric shocks, or being locked up in a cramped space.

Positive punishment Skinner was deemed to be unpleasant and reduced chances of being any thing

The event that preceded that will happen again like the smacking. Negative punishments are thought as the removal of something pleasant. It lowers the probability of positive response. Some examples include the removal of the money in your pocket; not watching television for the duration of a week.

It was Skinner"s study that determined the most effective method for altering behavior is by using the combination of punishing unacceptable behavior and positive reinforcement of desired behaviour.

Another type of psychological conditioning is called "operant conditioning". This type of training also has played a significant role in those who are type B. Operant conditioning can be used all the time in our efforts to influence others (type A personalities) or in another sense that people use it who influence us! As an example the parents or peers employ a complex and frequently unconsciously-designed program of punishments and rewards in order to motivate appropriate behaviour and deter inappropriate behavior.

It is important to talk about both kinds of conditioning because I believe they are related to Type B/A as well as B personalities. Every action that leads to the inhibition of emotions or thoughts within the person, according to my opinion, result in adverse effects for their health and it causes stress. The stress release of chemicals create a contraction in muscles and then the muscles that contract in consequently limit the flow of lymph and blood. This can be detrimental to our body since it eventually shuts down body"s organs, and in particular those of the lymphatic (immune) system.

The next publication will be Cooper"s version to the Bortner Type A scale, which was downloaded off the Internet (July 2005). The authors suggest that taking this survey will help to determine if you're an A or B personality. Mark an appropriate number for each one of the following statements to determine which one best describes how you act in daily day life. If, for instance, you generally showed up on time to appointments, then for the initial point, you'd mark a number that falls between 7-11. If you're more unobservant about appointments, you'd circle any number between 1 and 5. You can score your answers by adding the number of times you which you circled. Cooper"s assessment of your score can be described as the following:

The number of points you earn depends on the type of Person 85 or more Type A less than 84 Type B

Friedman along with Rosenman (1974) conducted studies into the reasons why certain people have a higher risk of suffering health issues due to stress than other people and how certain behavior patterns may act as warning signs of future illnesses. They studied the behavior patterns that sufferers of Coronary Heart Disease (CHD) and discovered that the same kinds of behaviour that kept appearing and they referred to them as the Types A behaviors.

The typical behavior of an A type person:

The thought of doing the same thing at the same time

Rushing to finish or rushing through your speech

Feeling extremely irritable when you are you are forced to stand in line

and driving in front of a vehicle or driving behind a car that you feel is going at a slow pace. You may notice knee or finger taps that are rapid and quick. and frequently using

obscenities

Being impatient when you watch others take actions

what you believe you are able to perform better or more quickly

Individuals who acted in an contrary way were called Type B behavior. A ten and half year research conducted by Rosenman (1975) revealed that people who were type A were twice as higher at risk of having heart attacks than people who had type B.

Eysenck"s (1985) The Theory of Neuroticism Dimension refers emotions in the personality of people, on one side of the spectrum were those who were calm and cool on the other hand were moody, temperamental individuals that were naturally fearful. The levels of emotional expression in a person could be classified into:

Socially acceptable Type of Extrovert Typical

Wants excitement

People to talk to Doesn't like party

Finds it difficult to stay entertained

Have many friends

Risks it all

Performs actions in a spontaneous manner

Easy and carefree Life and Soul of Party introvert Type B

Quiet

Introspective

Loves reading books

Reserved

Discovers amusement in his own friends take risks Rarely tends to think ahead and plan for the future Controls emotions

Steady/reliable.

A lot of research has been conducted in writing, published and extensively written about the negative impacts of stress on the body of people with person of the type A, which can lead to a higher risk of heart attacks, coronary artery disease and hypertension (hypertension) and more. This, as I"m certain we're aware, could be deadly.

While experts are well aware of the physical impacts to the body of a person being a Type A person but that they are not beginning to contemplate the consequences people with Type B personality traits could have.

It was a must!

There is a possibility of concluding by conducting research with individuals who have B/A or B

People with these traits may have issues in their lymphatic system. These types of personalities have the tendency of putting the needs of others" needs before their own. They are usually unable to say,,no" to the demands made on them, particularly from others and might struggle to convey appropriate emotions in the correct way to the individual. As an example, they may be able to have a tendency to complain about their friends however have not spoken towards the person who was the complaint was made. They are not averse to conflicts and prefer peace-lovers. My experience has shown that this kind of persona hides their real emotions, ensuring they remain inside, and displaying the appearance of a completely different emotions, or a façade. Because these feelings cannot be expressed, the feelings are internalized. It has been my experience that these inner feelings to be negative in their origin such as fear, anger, frustration and pain and anxiety. The negative emotions cause tension. The tension is manifested by tightening muscles. It is kept in that state over a long period of time and is shown, stop the lymphatic system from flowing, creating backflow that manifests in symptoms and signs.

In Summary

We are all aware of the effects of stress on people with type A or A/B personality. But, I do hope I've highlighted that those with type B/A or B personalities. They are also prone to serious health issues because they shut down the intensity of their emotions, and do not express them. that is known as internalisation. Certain experts believe that "bottling up things could cause serious harm to some kinds" and describes these as volcano"s ready to explode, clocking time bombs, whereas some say that putting things into" is similar to a cancer and consumes the person from within. Stress is a normal part of life situations; but what's more is it is that continual stress, emotional state can have detrimental effects on the body, organs and cells. are more susceptible to infections. In addition, so that the longer you are stressed, it's likely to cause negative effects upon the immunity system, ultimately which will have dire effects on the entire body.

Chapter 4: Methods Of Massage Used For The Sepia Technique

In this article, you'll discover the different massage techniques that are used in this technique. Sepia Technique. Although it's not required to master them, but it is important that you understand the basic principles at a fundamental level. As you begin using the Sepia Technique, you'll be uncertain about how you should apply pressure. The only thing I can tell you is that it will develop over the course of time as you gain the experience. As you practice the Technique the more adept you'll become with gauging the level of pressure that is required initially, however to begin it is likely that you choose to stay towards a lighter pressure. There will always there will be some discomfort as the areas being massaged are filled with painful waste and toxic substances. The common sense rule is the event that it becomes too uncomfortable, then ease down the pressure until less uncomfortable. Then, you can do it again a few days afterward. It can be beneficial to trim your nails small, because certain methods require a scooping or clawing motion by using your fingertips, so nails that are too long can rub against the skin, causing discomfort or irritation.

The method itself is broken down in two sections. Section 1" - the instructions for use with a partner and section ,,B" is the guidelines for self-administration. All methods must be followed applying a thick layer of oil, and apply massages to hair follicles. This will prevent the development of a condition referred to as Folliculitis (inflammation in the hair follicle, which is unpleasant). This chapter will help people to try how to massage in order in the Sepia Technique and the complete Sepia Technique instructions will be discussed in the following chapter this chapter.

The Sepia Technique Method

Instructions for A - Partner Massage Technique

1.) 1. Two-Finger Method diagram I

It is possible to use both hands in tandem or separately dependent on the size of an surface you're working with. For technique see next chapter.

Make sure to keep the fore and middle fingers in a row, then tuck your rest of your fingers in close proximity to your hand but not in the out of the way.

By using only the pads the fingers, press them into the skin.

After that, with consistent and even press against the tissues below, attempt to produce an sweeping stroke-like motion.

Begin at one end of the site node, keeping the pressure up until you get to the next end.

Remove your fingers from the area and continue this procedure until the areas have been massaged.

Diagram I

Take note that it isn't essential to use both hands at the same time. The alternation of your hands gives an even flow to the method and will allow for to even

the pressure of both hands for working the region (it can also be less demanding for hands because they're not under constant stress). Because the region you're doing work on is a node website, it is not a matter of what end you work at as long as the entire area of the space is fully covered.

2.) The Thumb over Thumb Massage Method (diagrams II and III)

For technique see next chapter.

Create a fist, and hold your thumb near it in order to shield your thumb from injury to ligaments (see the diagram I).

Only use the thumb pad to press hard on the fleshy region of the node's the site.

Begin at one end of the site for node, then move on to the next with short strokes of 25mm across the fleshy region.

Make sure you apply firm, equal pressure, but not so much that you be uneasy.

Alternate the thumb of the leader (the one on the front) for each stroke of 25mm, i.e. the thumb behind supporting will be the leader's thumb after 25mm. The one in front becomes the supporting thumb (behind

Diagram II

Keep the same amount of pressure each time you change your thumbs to ensure continuity.

This technique is extremely effective for solid lumps that are felt within the nodes to massage.

Diagram III

3) The Claw Massage Method (Diagram IV)

For technique see next chapter.

With your hands stretched out and fingers in a slack position, palms facing downwards form your hands to form downward-facing claws.

Using just the fingertips of your right hand beginning at the opposite end of the area where nodes are located and press the fingers down into the skin beneath as far as could be allowed.

Keep this firm, deep and firm pressure while moving your fingers over the node until you are at the other point of the node.

Remove the right hand. While at the same time, join to the left side (now made into a claw) in the beginning position.

Follow the steps above.

Keep alternating right and left until you have an effortless flow of movement until the entire area has been occupied.

The basic idea is to force as much into the area of flesh as can be tolerated by the patient who is receiving the Sepia Technique in order to squeeze all the contents from the lymph nodes. If the part which is treated appears to be bursting, the procedure may require two hands to create the shape of a claw (as as shown in the image above).

Diagram IV

4.) the Fist Massage Method (Diagram V) This technique is best applied to very tender areas just for

For instance, the armpits as well as behind the knees.

For technique see next chapter.

Make sure that all fingers form a fist. Tuck the thumb in.

near by, but not in easy reach.

Start at the edge of the node's location; Press the

Knuckle (first link that connects the fist) into the fleshy area. Maintaining the pressure for the duration of the entire process, use to create a

Sweeping or rolling action using your fist. Roll it across the surface towards the center, similar in rolling out

Pastry or kneading dough, but with your hands.

When you are done with the session, untie the hand.

Then, attach the 25mm in the direction to the right of the first

start point then repeat the process beginning point until you are

The entire area was covered.

It is not important whether you choose to use your right or left fist or even if you prefer to alternate between the left hand and then the right.

Diagram V

5) The Interlinked (double) Fist Massage Method (Diagram VI)

It is a complex method, and should be it is recommended to use only on large, bulky regions. For technique see next chapter.

Extend both hands out with fingers with palms facing downwards, with the thumb pointing toward the sides.

Join hands to slide your thumbs between palms. In this way, wrap your fingers in the thumbs (left hand grips the right thumb and right hand grips the left thumb). It is now time to start

With the flat end of your finger (not using the thumb) Press into the fleshy portion of the site for nodes to the depth that will be possible.

You can use a rolling or sweeping motion to the skin. This is as if rolling pastry.

Begin from the beginning of the node's side then work your way to the other

Remove the fists from their sockets, then connect at the beginning position so that you can begin the process again.

Diagram VI

This method might not be feasible for only one usage.

6.) 6. Scoop Massage Method (Diagrams VII and VIII) The method is intended exclusively for stomach problems.

For technique see next chapter.

Maintain your fingers in a straight line and joined. Use the pads of your fingers (to make sure there is that there are no

Nails are utilized) Bend your fingertips to the upwards, as high as possible for you to get the scooping motion.

With one hand only (e.g. left hand) Press down to the area that is fleshy in stomach, just below the ribs, and move towards your belly button.

The pressure needs to be firm enough to trigger a little discomfort. Make sure to maintain a consistent posture through the entire process to produce a solid glide.

Once you have reached the bellybutton, disconnect the right hand.

Join the left hand in the starting position then repeat.

Continue to alternate left hand with right until the whole sites of the node have been completely covered

Be aware that the amount of pressure that you will use is contingent upon the quantity of toxic substances present, the long they've been present and also your partner"s threshold to the toxins. However, as general rule of thumb, more tissue, the more pressure is necessary to reach the soft tissues.

Diagram VII

Diagram VIII

It is important to note that the technique operates best in the area where the nodes are located, it's necessary to push fairly deep. There are however only the soft, fleshy structures beneath which only include the womb and bladder as important organs, so women should take note of one of these periods that could be more sensitive during the moment, and thus you should ease the pressure during this period. This is especially true if you suffer from irritable bowel syndrome (although it is likely that once you've eliminated your lymphatics, this condition is going to be much better!) Furthermore, as this procedure touches the tip of these two structures, it might be beneficial before treatment to flush your bladder and the bowel, when you can. The "V" outline in image VIII is the location that needs to be treated.

The Sepia Technique Method

Instructions for B - Self Massage Technique

1) The Two Fingered Method (

Diagram I)

For technique see next chapter.

Create the fingers according to the instructions of your partner (A). If you're lying in a position with your head turned away from the place that you are working on, it will be difficult to perceive where you're doing your work, which is why it's important to become aware of the work you're doing.

While keeping both fingers to each other, put the pads of fingers in the site of the node from the beginning to near the ear.

The fingers should be pushed into the muscle behind the big muscles and drag the pads along the neck toward the chest in a gentle style.

You should maintain as much and consistent pressure as possible all the time.

At the point where you are at the bottom of the chest (nearest to the chest) take the fingers off and then reattach them towards the back, closest to the ear.

The other will follow" the previous one, and follow the same steps.

Diagram i

2.) The Two Fingered Method (diagram II)

For technique see next chapter.

Make use of the two fingers technique as in A for the groin nodes.

Diagram ii

3.) 3. The Thumb over Thumb Method (diagrams Iii and IV)

For technique see next chapter.

For this technique to be used on your own groin nodes, Follow the instructions for the procedure for

For use in the neck area, you'll have to move in upward motions through the chest towards the ear.

Diagram iii

Diagram iv

4.) A claw technique (diagram V)

For technique see next chapter.

Hands should be formed the same that you did for the A. The right hand to perform the left arm node (axilla) as well as the left hand to perform the right the axilla.

Begin at the base of the armpit. Press through the fleshy area of the armpit, and then pull the fingers all through the middle until they reach the chest area.

Repeat this procedure, shifting to the start position, which is 25mm counterclockwise for each stroke.

Keep a consistent pressure through each stroke.

Repeat the procedure until the space has been completely covered.

Diagram v

5.) Method of the Fist

(diagrams vi and diagrams vi and)

For you to successfully use this method for yourself, it is necessary to apply the right hand to the left side of your body as well as the left hand on the right side of your body for the exercise of underarms.

For technique see next chapter.

Make your hands into fists while keeping your thumbs on the outer of your fingers.

By using the knuckles you make a roll starting with the lower end (chest region) of the arm.

The knuckle is rolled as you are pressing into the fleshy region moving upwards toward the shoulder.

Repetition this procedure gradually around the entire area of the armpit to ensure that the armpit is being worked.

Self-administration using the Fist method.

Diagram vi

Diagram vii

6.) The scoop method to self (diagram VII)

In order to achieve the scoop technique for yourself, it's important to

Get yourself into the beginning position first (see Chapter 5). The depth of your treatment are able to achieve will be determined by the quantity of toxins that present in your region, the length of time they've been in there, and how much discomfort that you're willing to endure.

For technique see next chapter.

Start by using your thumbs and fingers extended straight, tightly to each other, hands in a downward direction.

You can achieve the scooping effect by rotating your fingers as far in the upward direction as you can.

Beginning at the left-hand outer border of the stomach, push the fingers of your left hand to the fleshy part of your stomach as far as you are able to comfortably.

Continue to apply this pressure while pushing your fingers downwards and away from you towards your belly button.

Keep the pressure constant throughout every stroke.

Take the left hand off and connect the right hand. Repeat the procedure.

Be sure to get comfortable with the movements using hands that alternate to make it an ongoing stream. The process will be a bit challenging but you'll get there eventually. It is important to note that this method is most effective at the depth the nodes are located, it is necessary to press quite deeply. There are however only subcutaneous soft tissues with just the womb and bladder as essential organs, so women take note of when you are going through a period and are more sensitive during the moment, which is why it's important to reduce the pressure during this period. Furthermore, as this technique touches the tips of these two structures, it is advisable prior to the treatment, to eliminate your bladder as well as your bowels if you are able to.

Diagram viii

Diagram depicts the disengagement of the right hand as well as the attachment of left hand.

6.) Reverse claw technique

Chapter 5: The Sepia Technique Before You Begin

To allow Sepia Technique to be effective, Sepia Technique to be effective ALL areas (node locations) require to be addressed with the same manner.

Oil- You can apply any oil that allows an spreading motion. For instance, arachis, baby oil, palm, olive corn, or vegetable oils. Make sure that the individual who is being treated for surgery isn't allergic or intolerant to the oil. It is possible to use the cream at a moderate rate, but be mindful of its drying qualities (see Gels).

Gels should not be used as they can cause friction on your skin (burns) in the event that they begin drying. In addition, they may cause skin irritation.

If it's your first time completed the treatment, be aware that the elimination of toxins stored in your body will undoubtedly have an impact on your body and you, therefore prepare yourself to take a break following the treatment. (also check out the post instructions for care below)

Following each treatment, it's important to flush out the body of toxins Therefore, it is advised to drink at a minimum of 2 liters of pure drinking water throughout the day in order to aid in this process and help neutralize the effects of.

Every treatment should be at least 48 hours between treatments so that the effects to diminish and for your body's immune system to adapt to the toxins that are stored.

In the aftermath of treatment, it can help in removing lymphatic system when you place your feet on the wall (see photo of leg elevation) for a period of 15 minutes.

The methods employed to perform Sepia Technique Sepia Technique require slow, intense pressure to be maintained throughout the process.

Be aware that the one negative indication against this method is when you are suffering from active cancer. That said if you are undergoing chemotherapy/radiotherapy for cancer, then the Sepia Technique can be most beneficial in clearing the debris caused by this treatment and also in boosting the immune system which is drastically depleted by chemo/radiotherapy regime.

Finally, the directions on Partner Sepia Technique will be identified as A. Likewise, instructions to SelfAdministration Sepia Technique will be indicated with a B. the procedure will be called S/T.

Preparation Instructions

With only your underwear on put a towel to rest your body on (to safeguard the flooring) of your sofa, couch or on the bed.

Place a small towel folded over or a pillow between your knees. You should have a pillow on your head on which to rest.

Bring a blanket or duvet for warmth and cover.

Place the couch or bed at a adequate height to allow the people who will be doing the procedure to ensure the correct posture.

It's not mandatory to play "mood" music however it does assist in relaxing, and contribute to a general atmosphere.

Instructions to use with the help of a partner (A)

A1- The Neck Nodes (Cervical)

I) Make your partner lie down on their backs. Do the same as you would for preparation.

II) Demand partner to turn their head towards the left

Iii) Finding the nodes. Then, ask your partners (in the same position) to raise their head. The neck's large muscle will reveal. The muscle to work across is all the way to the width of the space between the muscle with a width of about 25mm. The area in question is where cervical nodes reside.

IV) Apply oil to fingers and thumbs of the person doing the S/T. Apply on the cervical node.

V) Alternate with the method of two fingers and the thumb-over-thumb method for 3 minutes.

vi) Apply pressure to the neck as hard as is comfortable while keeping a steady, slow high pressure through.

A2- Neck Nodes (Cervical)

Ask the person with the S/T to rotate his or her head to the left after which repeat step Iii-Vi as described in A1 and then repeat it to the left side.

A3: A3 - Axillary Nodes (arm pits) Right arm) Invite your partner shift as much to the left end of the bed as far as is possible. As you do this, get your other person lying on the couch and bend the left arm until the elbow is at a level with the shoulder. The hand is resting on the head and palm pointing towards the upwards.

2.) You can ask your partner with a partner to apply oil on their fingers and apply it across the entire area of the armpits on the right side. If the hairs are particularly thick, you will require an extra amount of oil.

Iii) Apply the claw method as well as the single fist technique. Apply pressure to the area for 3 to 4 minutes. The more convex your area is, the greater depth it's required to be worked out, but it should remain within a it must be within the person"s area of

Always applying a consistent every stroke should be performed with a deep, even pressure. Iv) If the region is large or bulky, it's possible to employ double fisted technique (I have been able using this method)

A4: A4- Axillary Nodes- left arm

Switch to the opposite side, then repeat the steps to

A3 I- II, however in the pit on left side of arm

A5: The Abdominal Nodes (Cysterna Chyli) I) Wrap the shoulders in towels to keep them comfortable, revealing only the stomach region. Encourage your partner to bend the knees and keep the feet on the couch or bed and it is helpful to lift the head up slightly during this portion of the procedure, which allows the abdominal muscles to become completely in a relaxed state.

2.) Apply oil on the points of your hands. Spread the oil all over your abdomen region. Place your feet on the left of the massaged person with their backs to the feet.

II) The stomach area is divided into three areas including left side, centre and right side.

IV) Utilizing the scoop technique as well as the possibly thumb-over-thumb method to perform this method. Apply firm pressure into the soft tissue below. Please note that There aren't any bony structures there, and your body provides decent protection for all vital organs.

V) Begin from the outer edge of the rib that is on the left side of the stomach. Start with 10mm widths, and move 100-125mm length strokes toward your belly button/bikini line taking the line that runs under the rib cage. This is shown in the diagram VIII. You should slightly the strokes in between each one until you are at the center of the stomach. The process should take three minutes.

vi) If you are in the middle of your tummy (the hollow is referred to in the term solar plexus) Work over an area approximately 50 millimeters in width, then move between 100 and 125mm between the ribs to that belly button/bikini line an additional three minutes.

Vi) Transfer to the left side of the patient still standing with feet facing forward to repeat step iv V beginning with the outer part of the final rib located on the right side.

VIII) Reduce the knees, then take the upper body and cover it completely.

A6- The Groin Nodes (Inguinal)

1.) Make sure you are on the right-hand side of the individual facing their face and expose the right groin region.

II) The region to work on can be found when the knee is bent. there's a line across your knee (known as the Knicker Line) and you should work it for 20mm to either side of the line.

II) Request the person with the S/T put their left hand under the towel, and then pull the leg/underwear that is knicker-knifed to the left stomach (this allows the area which needs work as well as keeps their fingers clear of.)

IV) apply oil to the affected area.

(v) Utilize a mix of two fingers and the thumb-over-thumb method working on the region for about 3 minutes. This area could be extremely sensitive, so you must be aware and pay attention to your partner"s sensitivities and thresholds for pain.

vi) Apply a slow, firm and even pressure beginning at the outer edge of the leg. Work towards the inner leg (near the pubic bone).

VII) Do the work for three minutes.

VIII) Cover with a towels the groin region.

A7- The Groin Nodes (Inguinal)

I) Now, the partner moves towards the left and faces their partner.

II) Cover the left stomach. Request the person who is suffering from S/T to lay their left hand underneath the towel and keep their pants/knickers to the left side of their side of their groin (again it will reveal the area that needs to be treated)

Iii) Repetition steps iv-viii the same way as for A6, but with the left side of the groin.

A8 - Nodes at the Back of the Knee (popliteal)

I) remove the rolled-up towel from below the knees. Then ask your partners to flip over on their side. Make a double-fold of the rolled up towel and put it on the ankles or feet to raise the knees. Then, cover the body using towels or duvet.

I) Position yourself to the right side of the person who is facing their head. Remove the cover from the back of your right knee (known as the popliteal nodes)

Iii) The region that needs to be targeted is 25mm each along the entire length of the fold (seen in the rear of knee, when knee is bending downwards).

IV) Oil the surface to be worked

V) Utilizing the double fisted technique and alternatively, using the thumb over thumb technique to work over the entire region for at most 4 minutes.

vi) Cover the knee.

A9- Nodes at the Back of the Knee (popliteal)

1.) Go towards the opposite side of the bed. continue steps iii-vi for A8, but with a left knee.

Noting: Since the popliteal nodes tend to be the ones that are blocked, it could significantly enhance the efficacy of the Sepia Method if there was an additional massage is performed on the lower leg by gentle motions of the ankles toward the knee, to aid in the release of toxins that are stored in the body for another 4-minute session on each leg.

It is important to note that for those taking the treatment and those with knee problems and calves, or "cankles" (see photo on the next page). To maximize the benefits of the Sepia Technique it is recommended to be in the reverse position as illustrated on the following page for about 15 to 20 minutes per at night (preferably prior to going to bed as you'll then rest in a horizontal position, and not returning to your upright position, allowing the toxins to build up and then fill up again). In addition, due to the release fluids, lymph and toxins there may be a need to use your bathroom at evening.

Image showing a 70-degree elevation of the leg (note that knees have a slight bend and feet rest flat against the wall)

Image showing, "cankles"

(calves blend into ankles)

Self-Administration Procedures (B) Follow the steps to prepare as per instruction A for the partner. It is recommended to use nails that are very short as the majority of procedures require close contact with the fingertips.

B1- Neck Nodes (Cervical)

I) turn your head towards the left (to expose the left shoulder that is the back of your neck).

I) Then, in this posture, raise your head and feel the muscle which is being elevated. The region to work is directly behind the big muscle.

II) apply oil to the palms of both hands, and distribute the oil over the muscles behind them.

IV) Alternating both hands with the two-fingered approach, put the fingers down to the soft part of the ear between the ear and drag the fingers upwards until the point where neck meets shoulder.

•) Take the fingers off the hand. Attach them to the ear.

vi) Utilize one hand, with the other hand followed by the motion of stroking. Apply pressure as hard as you are able to and hold this level of pressure.

VII) Repeat the process. The area is worked for 3 minutes.

B2- Neck Nodes (Cervical)

I) Alternate to the other side i.e. move your head left (exposing the left side of your neck.

2.) apply oil on the palms of both hands.

II) Repetition steps iv-vii for B1.

B3- Axillary Nodes (armpit)

I) Transfer onto the right edge of the couch or bed.

I) 2. Take your left arm, turn the elbow in such a way that it's at a level shoulder. The armpit is visible and your hand is in front of the head. The palm is uppermost.

II) Apply oil using the right hand fingers.

IV) Utilizing the claw technique, Begin at the outside portion of the upper region in the armpit (near the shoulder) and push it in as hard and as far as you are able to, and then keep the pressure on and then drag your fingers towards the lower area (by between the ribs).

V) Repetition this motion taking 10mm off the start location in a counterclockwise direction and continue until you are about half way.

vi) In reverse, drag the fingers away from the area of the ribs towards the shoulder. Repeat 10mm increments, until the entire surface is filled.

Vi) Do this for about 3-4 mins.

Take note that armpits should be significantly swollen and full of toxic substances i.e. the armpits are bowed swelling, puffy or swollen apply the single fist technique using upward strokes (from the ribs up to the shoulder). Make use of the right hand to open in the left armpit. The reverse is also possible.

B4- Axillary Nodes

I) Make a shift to the left-hand end of the couch or bed.

II) bend the left arm until the elbow is at a level to the shoulder. the armpit of the right side is visible.

iii) Repeat steps B3 iii- vii

B5 - The Abdominal Nodes (Cysterna Chyli)

I) move to the centre of the couch or bed and then extend the knees, keeping the feet on the mattress. Make sure you are

Head rests on mattress

II) expose the stomach part, the tummy area is split into the left and middle, as well as the right side. We will perform all three.

Iii) The location is at the bottom of your ribs on the left side of your tummy. the work will go down the ribcage until you reach the opposite side (see diagram VII). Each movement will go downwards until your belly button (umbilicus).

IV) Apply oil on the palms of both hands.

V) The scoop method is the scoop method using two hands, alternating strokes using each hand.

vi) Begin on the left side of the ribcage (see diagram V) Push down the tummy's fleshy region stomach with your left hand.

Vi) Keep this pressure in place as you push towards your belly button.

VII) As you remove your left hand from the belly button, place the right hand in the position you started from as you repeat steps vi and vii.

IX) Repeat the pattern shifting 10mm every time you move toward the middle. This will take about 3 minutes.

x) The middle (the hollow in which the right rib join the left) employ the technique of the overlap scoop to create an area 20mm to either from the middle for an additional three minutes.

(xi) Then repeat the exercise for the opposite part of the ribs. Make sure to use your right hand as the lead hand and repeating steps iv-IX.

B6- The Groin Nodes (Inguinal)

I) This is the part where you might find it comfortable to take off your pants since it is the self

administration. Put a cushion under your knees and gently lift them. This will relieve away the stress on the area of the groin node.

II) Remove the right groin in a way that you can keep all the other members of your body warm.

III) Apply the oil on the palms of the hands (copious amounts, if the region around the groin is full of hair).

IV) The region is located when bending the knee. A wrinkle can be seen at the upper part of the leg. the work area will be 25mm along across the entire length of this crease.

(v) Make use of a mixture of two fingers and the thumb-over-thumb method moving 10mm segments along the length.

vi) Apply firm pressure that starts from the outer skin of the leg. Then move towards the inside of the of the leg (near the pubic bone). Be aware that this region can be very sensitive. Be aware about the amount of pressure you exert (stay within your personal tolerance to pain).

VII) Apply pressure to the entire area for three minutes. Try to work the same as hair growth in order to prevent the folliculitis (inflammation in the hair follicle)

VIII) Find the part of the groin.

B7- The Groin Nodes (Inguinal)

I) Remove the left groin then repeat steps iii-viii with the right groin.

B8 - Nodes at the Back of the Knee (popliteal)

To do this, you'll have to lay on the bed, and your head towards the end of your foot and your feet with your back flat on the wall, with knees bent or lying on your floor with a towel with your feet resting flat against the wall (as as per the picture that shows the leg's elevation to 70 °). The top of your body should be covered in order to stay warm. lay a cushion under your head.

The image shows how to clear the node in the popliteal region by auto-administration Sepia Technique.

1.) apply oil on the palms of both hands.

I) Begin with the left popliteal node. The area which needs to be addressed is approximately 25mm to either side of leg's crease; do the entire length of the crease.

III) It is the reverse claw technique (see the image on the following page). Make your hands into claws and then turn your hands to make sure that your fingers are facing you. The right hand is performing the work behind your knee on to the right, while the left hand is doing the same work on the left.

Iv) Join the fingers of your right hand on the space 25mm over the knee crease and 25mm in front of the knee (again look at the picture on the following page).

Chapter 6: How Can You Tell If The Lymphatics In Your Body Are Blockage?

This section is meant to provide you with a brief overview indicators and signs that I have observed through my study. If, when you go through the short check-list below, you can answer "yes" to at least four of the symptoms and signs and symptoms, then it's likely the lymphatic system in your body isn't working exactly as it ought to. Therefore, it makes sense to conclude that your lymphatic system is not functioning properly. The more symptoms that you are able to identify with the more deterioration is in your lymphatic system. Look around and determine the number of people you can recognize with.

Quick Test Guide

Look through the below list to determine if your lymphatics are blockage. If you can answer "yes" in more than four of them, then you'll surely benefit from Sepia Technique. Sepia Technique.

Are you a Type B or BA person? (See chapter 3.) Are you working an occupation that is sedentary, where you standing or sitting down often? Are you suffering from one or more of the following?

Are you a victim of tension for an extended period of duration of time during the past or currently?

Physiological Signs and Symptoms

Legs that are aching

Asthma/wheeziness/breathlessness

Abdomen that is inflamed/bloated

Bowel disorders e.g. IBS, constipation, flatulence. Calf and ankles meet but without specificity

Circulatory problems- extreme cold, discoloration of the limbs, numbness or sensations of tingling e.g. carpal tunnel signsbleeding gums or pain and constant toothache.

Disturbed sleep

Eye irritations such as conjunctivitis or sticky eyes.

Exhaustion

Flu-like symptoms

Gastro-intestinal disturbances e.g indigestion, trapped wind, dyspepsia

General malaise

Headache/Migraines

Heavy leg syndrome

Musclestight, squeezed, cramping

Menopausal symptoms (all)

Acute ailments like frequent coughs, sore throats or colds.

Verrucae, boils, warts Herpes (cold sores)

Numbness- In limbs, fingers, toes

Unexplained pain - nowhere

Skin texture that is tight or rubbery (see the pictures A and B in the introduction chapter)

Swollen joints

Skin complaints e.g. pruritus, eczema (itchiness) or acne dry skin with flaky texture or the psoriasis (stressed by stress)

Sinusitis, sinus troubles

The neck is stiff and incapable of turning head in the right direction in order to view the other side of the person behind you

while reversing a vehicle

Swelling (oedema) It can occur anywhere, however especially in the stomach wrists, but also in the tummy

lower limbs.

Tinnitus or ear infections.

Tonsillitis and throat troubles

Legs twitching

Watery/Dry eyes/conjunctivitis

The weight gain is most noticeable at the midriff

Complicated Ailments

Chronic Fatigue Syndrome

Glandular fever

Leg Ulcers and those are not healing or responding to treatments

M.E.

M.R.S.A/ C. Diff

Neutropenia

The post-operative complications/not getting properly

Post Chemo/Radio Therapy Regime

Systemic Lupus Erythematosus (SLE)

Toxoplasmosis

Psychological Signs and Symptoms

The uncontrollable cry of the children

Depression (excluding those with a clinical diagnosis of depression)

I. because of discomfort

ii. because of trauma

iii. because of situations

Judgemental errors

Lethargy

Lack of Energy

Insufficiency of motivation

Low Libido (sex drive)

Self-esteem is low.

Changes in mood

Nervousness/anxiety

Peer Pressured

Phobias were recently discovered.

Refrain from social or other groups

Chapter 7: Maintaining Your System

Amazing as the Sepia Technique results are at restoring your quality of life; ridding you of those minor/major ailments that invaded your body conditionsyou were told to ,,learn to live with;" giving you back your long lost energy levels; it is important to remember that you may need to look at making some changes in your lifestyle/circumstances to prevent your lymphatic system becoming re blocked. This chapter is aimed at ways of helping you maintain your body now it has been restored.

The Sepia Technique is a procedure that can repeated for as many times as possible. You should to allow the treatment for 48 hours to overcome the post calculation that results from the release of toxic substances. This would be the perfect moment to tell you about the potential could happen as a result of the aftermath. If your nerves are restricted, which is when your skin appears rigid and difficult to move; you show a variety of indicators and signs, or if your node sites appear convex, then it is possible to think that, after the first session of The Sepia Technique you are likely to experience more effects than those who show just a handful of indications and symptoms. Before we examine the possible outcomes following the Sepia Technique to treat you, we must start by determining the reason we experience them. The answer may be intuitive to many that when you've got toxic waste and waste products (poisonous substances that can be harmful to your wellbeing) which are within the body, hidden and secured by your nodes and the nodes themselves, it makes sense that should they to enter the body, they would eventually trigger reactions. Although this reaction is only temporary lasts for around 24 hours while the body is able to eliminate the toxins, can be manifested as the following: one, two or (if the lymph nodes of your body are constricted) additional of the following:

stool that is loose

Strong and/or strong-smelling Urine headaches that are dark in colour

nausea (and occasionally vomiting)

pimples, spots (and occasionally, boils)

general malaise, feeling "under the weather"/flu similar to

the symptoms

Feeling cold and shaking

The above adverse symptoms have been mentioned by a few of my patients prior to their therapy. But let me tell you right away that the side consequences were significantly reduced when the diluting of them using water (see the following points). The more treatment sessions you have, the lesser the adverse negative effects (assuming that you're not reviving them by replacing the causes," and you are not sustaining the current condition!) in addition you are likely to notice the symptoms and signs get less. Thus, it's beneficial for your mental health by making an exhaustive list of symptoms and signs before beginning using the Sepia Technique and periodically check this list to observe how the situation has changed. In the example above, if prior to when you began, you had headaches, write this down however, note how frequently you experience them, and the grades they fall into and the length of time they will are lasting, and as you go back, you will be able to see how things have improved, meaning that it is possible that you still suffer from headaches, but they're smaller and less painful and don"t take as long to heal, etc, (whereas the brain tells it that you're suffering from headaches!)

For maximum benefit, you need cleanse all of the lymph nodes from all the toxic substances, and then continue to maintain the system and alter the habits that resulted in the system being restricted. When it has happened because the symptoms and signs from the list of symptoms (see chapter 6.) will reverse, which is, they'll have drastically decreased or disappeared completely.

Additionally, you'll recognize when you require a top up" Sepia Technique since your body's signals will tell you when it's time. This is the only way you will have the ability to notice and do something about it right away! Don't allow it to spiral back into the condition you first started the technique in.

There are a variety of factors you should consider after you've cleansed your lymphatic system.

Considerations

Take care to address the stressors in your life: Finda ,,relief technique," for example, physical exercise releases the chemical adrenalin that gives us a ,,lift," meditation may allow you to contemplate the difficult times you've faced and also think "outside the box" so that you can come up with a solution. It could also be beneficial to sit down and find a sense of peace that you did not know existed or had the ability to achieve. Going to outdoor activities is sure to get your mind off tension, so make sure you choose an activity or class that you like and is both challenging and satisfying for your. There are a lot of self-help resources and sites to offer solutions for your anxiety however, I recommend you attempt to address your stress's root causeand this could mean looking for help from professionals or more in-depth

Life circumstances can be a drastic change however if this was the reason for many problems, maybeit"s the time to re look at.

The things you do can cause the blockage to block it. Perhaps your work involves a lot of sitting or standing. This causes the lymphatics to accumulate and the node that is the furthest from your main drainage i.e. those located on the back of the knee are initially affected. The people who live this type of lifestyle/job that requires a lot of sitting must be encouraged to move regularly" This could mean that you take an easy 20 minutes walk during your lunch break. You can also choose to walk instead of the lift and make sure you are elevating your foot at 70 degree mark!

If you feel that your stress levels have gotten out of control (the boss is putting more and greater requirements on you) it might be a good idea to consider taking assertiveness courses to understand how to respond with "no" when 5 minutes before you are due to go home he/she wants that letter typed and in the post today! Look up" broken record method" It's very helpfulbegin by practicing for someone near you to increase confidence. Then bite the bullet and watch the results-you might surprise yourself.

Stress can come in it's form as pressure placed on your body by many ways, not only psychological. Find a way to lessen the amount of stress your body is forced to bear on a regular schedule, however uncomfortable it may be, it's essential that you and your brain are allowed to relaxation" to cleanse it of any contaminants and build its immunity levels. It is essential to sleep for this reason, therefore make sure just before the time you go to bed, you are able to relax

For instance, it's not worth doing a crossword game at night; if it is not completed, you'll take the unfinished words along with you, and toss and turn throughout the evening; watching news and becoming upset by what you see can play in your head all night long and thinking about the things you'll need to complete the next day will keep you from getting a complete sleepI suggest you create a checklist to ensure that your brain is able to shut down and you will be able to rest assured that you won"t be able to remember anything. TipKeep the list in your pocket to use in the event that one of those tiny demons that have gone unnoticed pops into your thoughts during the night and you decide to add it to the list, and return to sleep.

Create your own "time" at the end of the day to unwind, take a bath, read a novel, listen to relaxing music you enjoy. Avoid coffee last thing at all costs- it is a stimulant as well as a diuretic and will dehydrate your body. It is vital in this incredibly fast world we live in to „slow down" and let your body to heal.

Don"t workout before bedtime aside from the release of adrenalin that gives you an "lift" the body generates waste products or acids detrimental to your body. They are unable to be absorbed by your body because you are resting, and, as we know, that the lymphatic system relies on muscles' action to circulate it around your body.

If you're doing any exercise, be sure to are warming up before winding down! Your wind-down should consist of stretches for a long time that remove toxins that are produced through muscles, and don"t not forget to turn your legs by bending them at 70 degrees for the drainage. Trust me when I say that you'll be able to feel the speed with which the legs will be able to recover.

Diet. Yes, the fearful word can be used to describe this. It also impacts on your immune system. Simple carbohydrates have small nutritional value yet are a plethora of calories, for instance cake, pastry, crisps/nibbles refined white bread (cheap white) sweets, biscuits. The effect is offer the body the ability to quickly fix itself, making it feel" and act more alert for a very short time, but what goes up must come down. The affects are very short lived, making you feel ,,low" and you then reach to get more of the stuff that gives you that boost and the cycle continues.

The only issue is that the foods they are high in calories that the amount you consume exceeds the amount you consume, which results in weight gain! Furthermore, the large quantity of carbohydrates means you body"s metabolism is occupied trying to breakdown these foods into fat that is stored (nice one) which drains the body, causing levels of energy to decrease and you feel drained. Be mindful of these kinds of foods and keep it in the fridge for events that are only for special occasions and try to avoid eating the "bad foods" in the morning before eating lunch to ensure you're able to "burn off the calories." Do not eat simple carbohydrates at late at night as you'll get energized through its effects and cause insomnia.

Make sure you drink more water. It's not easy to do if you're not used to drinking water, but trust me, you'll eventually enjoy drinking it. Take a look at it this way: water isn't a source of nutrition or calories and therefore serves as a flush to the lymphatic system. Furthermore, because it is clean and clean, it is a pure fluid, and the body"s immune system doesn't require any processing which is why it doesn't help in preventing the body from working. Start by substituting 1 cup of coffee or tea for drinking a glass of pure water every day. You can gradually increase it to two glasses in a week, and so up to. Keep in mind that 70 percent of your body is from water. Every cells in your body require water in order to function.

Chapter 8: What Is The Lymphatic System?

The lymphatic system is component of the circulatory system comprised of the conduit networks. They are referred to as lymphatic vessels. These vessels carry clear fluid to the heart. Thomas Bartholin and Olaus Rudbeck were the first to describe this method in the 17th century. Contrary to what is commonly believed it isn't an isolated system. Actually, it is a system that works in conjunction with blood vessels as well as the heart in order to return a substantial amount of the liquid that has been lost in the blood circulation. This way it allows your body to ensure that electrolytes are in balance through the process of the process of fluid homeostasis within the body.

Lymph

The lymph fluid is the one that circulates through the veins within the system. It is an equivalent to the circulation system's blood. The liquid involved in the transport of white blood cells as well as other related immune system elements. In essence, lymph also consists of large amounts of plasma as well as other liquid components from the blood.

Lymph Nodes

Lymph nodes are arranged collections of lymphoid tissues that the lymph flows through prior to when returning to the blood flow that is main. They can be found across the whole lymphatic system. The lymph node's components have a lot in common with the organs of kidneys. The lymph nodes are typically made up of: (1) cortex; (2) Medulla; as well as (3) hilum. A number of lymph vessels afferent to the brain can draw in lymph, which moves into the interior of lymph nodes. The lymphatic fluid is then flushed through the lymph vessels that are efferent.

Spleen

The most significant lymphatic organs includes the spleen. This assists with the process of processing lymphocytes after lymph and blood separate from the circulatory system that is distal. It is a soft, sponge-like organ, approximately the size of the size of a fist. In terms of anatomy, it is situated on the left side in the abdominal area. This area is directly under the ribcage. Apart from the processing aspect, this could also aid in the decomposition of blood vessels to facilitate excretion.

Mucosal Lymphatic Tissues

The mucosal lymphatic tissues can be tissues that are able to acquire antigens via transcytosis into the lymphoid tissue. Antigens are blood constituents that help to establish protection in case the body is contacted by a foreign object. This means that these tissues could aid in establishing a strong defence mechanism, with an in-built memory of the characteristics of the foreign body which infiltrates your system. This allows the body to counteract harmful results of the foreign body in the event that it ever is introduced into the system.

WBC's

They are also referred to by the name of white blood cells. They are the major blood-borne components which help to promote an improved immune system.

They work in tandem to assist in the restoration of balance within the body. Understanding the way these components function can assist you in understanding how the body operates on the larger scale. This can assist you in understanding how lymphatic system disorders affect the body. Based on these principles, knowing the fundamental elements of the system will help you understand the treatments.

Chapter 9: How The Lymphatic System Works

The lymphatic system does not only a network of vessels and nodes filled with fluids that move through the body. In this article we will provide more information details about the way that lymphatic systems work to assist your body's function more effectively. Understanding how the system functions can assist you in determining the best way to utilize the body's voluntary organs in order to assist the lymphatic system's parts work more efficiently. Apart from that, the information can assist you in coming with proactive measures to keep your lymphatic system safe from possible disorders.

Transportation and Collection

The primary purpose of the body system is to carry and store the tissues fluids that transport. The fluids that transport tissues typically are derived from intracellular space. These intracellular space, which are in turn, can be located in a majority of tissues of the body. When the fluids have been brought into these areas, the system is then able to bring those fluids back to your circulation system via the veins.

Plasma Protein Return

The lymphatic system plays an crucial roles with regard to the transfer of plasma proteins back into the bloodstream. It is crucial because plasma proteins include blood elements that play a significant role in healing wounds as well as renewal of the skin layer. The reason for this is that plasma proteins are a source of ingredients that help to produce reinforcement agents that help slow the process of bleeding. The substances also aid in helping to create a temporary layer which will help to stop the entry of additional foreign substances in your body.

Fat Processing

The body also can absorb fats and digest them via lymphatic systems. Once digested and absorbed the lymphatic system helps in transferring them to the small intestine, and the bloodstream through the villi. The small intestines make use of the lacteals as well as the lymph vessels to facilitate efficient transport of fats and other substances to various regions in your body.

Lymphocyte Production

The lymph nodes play a role for the creation of lymphocytes. They will take over the lymphocytes of old that are set to be removed out of the body. The production of a fresh batch of lymphocytes can help in increasing the efficiency that the immune system. This helps the body to fight off ailments that could affect many tissues and organs.

Immune System Buildup

This is in line with the lymphatic system is accountable for aiding the body to continuously boost its defense system body. This is done through the production of substances by enzymes which allow the body to remember the characteristics of the foreign organism that may attack the body in the near future. Experts use the same idea for both the creation as well as the creation of vaccines. They are the substances that assist you in avoiding contracting an illness that is serious by providing their less hazardous alternative.

At the time that this article was written, researchers are conducting research in order to better understand the functions that could be performed by the lymphatic system. Learning more about the function of the lymphatic system will assist them in understanding the benefits each component in the system could bring. Long-term it can be a huge factor to the efficient diagnosis and the treatment of disorders affecting lymphatics.

Chapter 10: Common Lymphatic System Disorders And Diseases

The lymphatic system usually experiences various issues which impact not just the lymphatic system but also different body system. It is particularly evident with cancers in the majority of cases. If the cause of cancer persists undiagnosed for long periods and the lab results be most likely to indicate that the person affected suffers from a disorder of the lymphatic system. It is often referred to as metastasis. It can also contribute to the spread of cancerous cells as the lymphatic system usually covers all of the body's organ tissues.

Lymphoma

Lymphoma is a disease of the body, which manifests via rapidly growing lymphocytes with malignant characteristics that can last over long time. They accumulate in lymph nodes and different lymphatic system areas and, eventually, form cancerous tumors. If they are found to accumulate in lymph nodes, they're commonly referred to as Adenopathy. The majority of the time, this is recognized due to the swelling of lymph nodes. The cause of Adenopathies can be different including poor health, or genetic causes.

Hodgkin's Lymphoma

Hodgkin's Lymphoma could be thought of as a variant of the disease previously mentioned. It is a type of cancer which is most often found within the lymph nodes. The diagnosis of this condition can be determined in a different way based on the development of tumorous tissue during biopsies. The most common Hodgkin's Lymphoma and the NLPHL or nodularly derived Hodgkin's lymphoma that is primarily a lymphocyte. Similar to the other cancerous disorders, the disease is manifested through the signs and symptoms that include: (1) Weight loss; (2) Profuse sweating at night; (3) Severe itching across the body, mainly those on the legs. (4) breathing problems (5) dry cough; (6) fever; (7) Unexplained fatigue or fatigue; and (8) painless and large lymph nodes, which feel rubbery when you touch them.

Non-Hodgkin's Lymphoma

Non-Hodgkin's Lymphoma can also be an incurable condition that affects the lymphoid organ system. The disease is further subdivided into three types: (1) intermediate grade; (2) low grade and (3) the highest grade. Of these three kinds three, the last one is the most rapid-growing type. If it is not addressed, this may even put a strain on the health of the patient suffering from the illness. However the type with the lowest grade tends to be the least likely to manifest. It is not likely to show symptoms or signs immediately. As opposed to the more severe form, this type of cancer cannot be managed with one of the cancer-related treatments of the lymphoid system.

Lymphadenopathy

Lymphadenopathy is a disease which typically manifests as the swelling of multiple lymph nodes. It can be confined only to certain lymph nodes. However it is possible that the swelling could be widespread. Based on this, the severity of the problem is a major factor in the severity of the disease. This means that the more severe form of lymphadenopathy could cause the condition to progress throughout the bloodstream. If the problem is localized, the primary cause could be due to foreign particles, infections or other issues located within the lymph vessels, and lymph nodes. The nodes with inflammation due to infections can cause pain on contact. However swelling nodes due to cancerous cells tend to be painless.

Chapter 11: Treatment Options

To reap the benefits from a suitable program for treatment to treat a particular lymphatic system problem it is essential to know about the correct diagnosis procedures you have to go through. This is essential because it could help medical professionals discover the specific condition you suffer from. The proper diagnosis of the condition can assist doctors create an individual and precise treatment program that will assist in addressing all the difficulties you experience due to the condition.

Internal Examination

There are various areas that require a more thorough examination since the lymph nodes typically are close to or in proximity to the main organs. In the beginning, experts have to check the lymph nodes in the body. The lymph nodes are located in the abdomen and thoracic cavity. They're difficult to detect. Furthermore, their growth will not be seen in blood samples that are routinely taken. They can, however, be evident on radiographs or ultrasound examinations when they've been excessively enlarged. Experts can also be able to detect them through exploratory surgical procedure. The sternal lymphoid nodes and the mesenteric lymphnodes could be detected using these techniques.

Palpation

However there are other lymph nodes could be located by the use of palpation. The only thing the doctor needs to do is press the area of concern using the pads of fingers. It is essential to apply firm pressure in order to ensure that they are able to detect the lymph node clearly. Here are a few lymph nodes that can be easily felt:

The prescapular lymph node can be situated just behind the shoulder area. In order to locate this node, follow the arm until the point at which you shoulder.

Submandibular nodes are located within the neck area. The node lies at the angle of your jaw. Since they're located near the salivary glands of your mouth and salivary glands, it can be somewhat difficult to find the.

Inguinal lymph nodes could be found near the abdomen. In particular, they may be situated within the medial areas of the legs. The fat may be through the feeling. This is why you might need to work harder against the region.

It is the easiest for you to locate these popliteal nodes. They're usually found in the rear of the knees.

Aspiration

Another way to diagnose is to use fine needle aspiration. To perform this procedure an examiner must employ a needle that is fine and then gently place the needle onto the lymph node that is suspected to be. Following this, the specialist will remove a small amount of lymph node from it and put it in a microscope for examination. To conduct the proper examination the sample is placed onto a microscope slide for additional examination.

The pathologist will place an appropriate stain on the lymph. The findings will be determined by the response of the lymph in response to the dye.

Biopsy

The most popular techniques for diagnosing is using the biopsy. It requires an examiner to remove the whole lymph node, and then place the area under a microscope to allow more detailed examination. As opposed to the aspiration technique it can give additional information about the exact nature of the lymphatic system issue.

In the previous section, a variety of diseases of the lymphatic system were described. Diagnostics usually go together with specific treatment. This section is specifically dedicated to discussing the particular treatments that can be used for these ailments. Other treatment options for different ailments are covered in this section. Understanding the various treatments that could be utilized for these ailments could help doctors and patient determine the best plan of treatment that will precisely address the symptoms and signs sufferers are experiencing.

Lymphoma

Treatment for lymphoma depends on the amount of radiation therapy and chemotherapy. The stage at which the patient is in their cancer can influence the decision-making. Although there are many variables that determine the best treatment plan to be utilized, the primary and second stage of the disease are generally managed with radiation treatment. In the case of more severe cases chemotherapy may be recommended. In certain cases it is possible to use adjuvant therapy employed. Particularly if the patient is in the remission stage.

Hodgkin's and Non-Hodgkin's Lymphoma

Treatment of Non-Hodgkin's as well as Hodgkin's Ly is basically the same. Similar to the treatment for lymphoma treatment, the strategy of treatment will depend on the present stage of the disease. Naturally, lower grades of cancers can be managed by using the less invasive methods. The majority of them can be treated by a single procedure. In contrast high-grades may need an array of treatments to deal with the issue. Furthermore, certain circumstances such as the presence of additional conditions may influence the treatment as well as the kinds of medicines that are used to treat the sufferer. Below are a few alternatives to treatment that can be considered to treat these ailments: (1) monoclonial antibody therapy; (2) radiation therapy; (3) autologous stem cell transplantation as well as (4) chemotherapy.

Lymphangitis

Another issue that can be managed using medication is called lymphangitis. The treatment is generally antibiotics. The early diagnosis of this issue as it can identify if doctors need take other measures to prevent the risk of spreading infection to the bloodstream. Alternative methods employed to treat the condition are regular bandaging, and the drainage of lymphatic fluids through cutting the region. It is generally used when the affected area is a upper or lower part of the extremity.

Lymphangiectasia

In the case of lymphangiectasia treatment, the method that is chosen should be targeted at the signs and symptoms. If the type is intestinal that is the most common type, treatment tends to be geared toward changing the diet. Particularly, the nutritionist or dietician can suggest food foods that are rich in fatty acids. These contain medium chains. Additionally, a low-fat diet is suggested. For further relief from symptoms and signs, your doctor may also prescribe remedies to stop diarrhea. The majority of them are utilized to ease stomach pain and improve the motility of the stomach as well as the intestinal tract.

Lymphatic Filariasis

Oral Albendazole and Diethylcarbamazine citrate and Ivermectin are commonly used to treat lymphatic filariasis. They are usually employed to eliminate the nematodes that inhabit the area. In order to prevent prevention of future outbreaks, mosquito control is the only method that works.

Chapter 12: Preventive Measures

One of the most popular doctors who deal with lymphatic system concerns are physiotherapists. They typically assist by employing the use of electrical, mechanical and thermal techniques to assist patients reduce symptoms and signs that they may experience due to their illness. In this section we will provide you with more information about the particular methods specialists employ to lower the risk of lymphatic system issues and treat the symptoms and symptoms that might pop out. They can also be employed in order to protect you from problems related to the lymph system.

Considerations

Keep in mind that the effectiveness of the treatment of lymphedema will primarily be determined by the overall circulation of lymph as well as the structures in nature that could be situated near the affected region. The area affected for drainage will help identify what specific patterns the physiotherapist could use for manually drained lymphatic drainage. Additionally, it can help if self-massage is to be used to treat the problem.

Self-Massage and Manual Lymph Drainage

The possibility of performing self-massage or manual lymph drainage. These could be achieved through stimulation of the lymphatic vessels between the large lymphatic vessels and at the end. They can aid in stimulating the lymphatic flow within the system. This can also aid in opening up the area to allow lymphatic fluids to get into the capillaries when the treatment continues. The treatment will continue with the help by gentle massaging. This method aids in stimulating the flow of excess lymph within the areas affected. The movements for massage must be gentle and steady in order to provide the proper quantity of tension. This is crucial for the effective flow of lymph through the capillaries.

Compression Garments

Another approach to lessen swelling and inflammation due to lymph system issues is by using compression clothing. They are cloth pieces which resemble stockings. They are, however, different from the standard clothing, they are graded in accordance with the amount of pressure they put on the surface that they will be used. These compression clothing are generally utilized for mild cases. If not, tighter compression clothing are employed.

Exercises

Training and active movement exercises are essential in transferring the excess lymph across the body from one location to the other. In these techniques muscles of the major groups can be the most effective devices that are able to help get the fluid moving in the right direction. The trampoline is a great tool to do well in stopping the development of issues with lymphatics. It is particularly effective when you consume lemon water regularly on daily basis. daily routine. In order to further enhance the flow of lymph, specialists suggest that patients put on compression stockings during exercises. Utilizing free weights can help in boosting the force of the muscles exertion to bring lymph into the capillaries.

Patients should be active to manage their ailments. This is essential as they'll have to practice the techniques on a regular schedule. That is among the main reasons why physiotherapists frequently use these techniques as a at-home program for patients. In addition to helping patients and their families develop confidence and a proactive approach to taking care of the disease the home-based program could aid them to become more confident in dealing with their actual situation.

Chapter 13: Related Topics

Apart from the fundamental elements, there are many different stages of development that must be understood regarding the lymphatic system goes. In this section you'll learn the process of development of lymphatic tissue. This knowledge can assist you to discover how conditions develop in the body system. This knowledge can assist you develop a more efficient plan of treatment with your doctor should you need to go through physiotherapy or medical strategies to deal with your present health issue. Additionally, it can help to identify early signs of problems in pregnancy.

Pregnancy

The lymphatic tissues begin developing at the end in the 2nd month in the embryonic stage. The lymphatic vessels develop from lymph sacs, which are formed from the circulation system's veins. They originate from mesoderm. The mesoderm has been regarded as one of the earliest precursors of the nervous system. In addition to these components there are other branches of the lymphatic system are created from this fundamental part of the nervous system.

Jugular Lymph Sacs

The initial batch of lymph sacs which come out are the pair of Jugular lymph sacs. They can be found near the cross-section of the subclavian as well as the internal Jugular veins. In the lymph sacs that are located in the jugular zone, capillaries of lymphatics expand to the trunk the neck, head as well as the upper extremities. Certain plexuses expand and form lymphatic vessels within their respective areas. Every jugular lymph sacs is home to at least one connection to the base jugular vein. The left-hand portion develops towards the superior end of the Thoracic duct.

Retroperitoneal Lymph Sac

The second of the lymph sacs which appear is the retroperitoneal lymph sac. It is an unpaired lymph sac, which is situated on mesentery's root within the intestinal tract. It is formed by the mesonephric veins, as well as the primitive Vena Cava. The lymphatic vessels, as well as capillary plexuses are then able to spread out into the retroperitoneal lymph sac in order to further spread into the diaphragm as well as abdomen viscera. The lymph sac is then able to create connections to the cistern and chyli. But, these connections are eventually lost due to the presence of the veins in neighboring veins.

Posterior Lymph Sac

The lymph sacs in the posterior region follow in the development of posterior lymph sacs. The paired sacs originate by the vessels of the iliac. The lymph sacs are the capillary plexuses and lymphatic vessels that are located in abdominal walls, in the lower legs, as well as the within the pelvic area. They are linked to the cerebellar the chyli. They cease to be connected to nearby veins of the circulatory system.

Lymphatic Invasion

Each of the lymph sacs which develop are infiltrated by mesenchymal cells. A notable exception of the posterior lymph sac. The infected areas are converted into various groups of lymph nodes.

Once the formation in the lymphatic system slows to an end and the lymphatic system is unable to function, it will begin functioning by collaborating with the circulatory system in order to provide effective extraction and recirculation fluids. Over time this will aid in maintaining the electrolyte and fluid balance throughout the body. In addition, it could aid in the efficient elimination of fluids your body doesn't require any more.

Chapter 14: Lymphoid Organs

Primary Lymphoid Organs:

Bone Thymus and Marrow

The embryos appear early in life

The lymphocyte-specific site of education identify self and nonself antigens Immune competence

The pathways are not a part that allow for antigen penetration.

1.Bone Marrow :

The red marrow is active and hemotopoietic as well as the inactive and fatty yellow Marrow.

The bone marrow serves as the place for B lymphopoiesis.

The bursa of the Fabricius site of differentiation and generation of LB (its removal is a source of trouble of humoral immune system only) different from LT cells.

2.Thymus :

It ends its organogenesis in the 20th week. The maximum size is in puberty (adolescent)

The site of LT maturation and differentiation

Cortex: immature LT + feeder cells

Medulla adult LT and epithelial cells (Hassal's corpuscle) + dendritic cells, and macrophages (IL-1)

Thymocytes are subject to a double selection:

Positive: corticomedullary area: Thymocytes that detect the peptide-CMH pairing are able to receive an indicator of survival

Negative: medullary area Thymocytes that express the TCR receptor with very high affinity to self peptides are removed. Self peptides are removed.

II.Secondary lymphoid organs

Later, later development that is located along the channels of the penetration of antigens

Symbiotic: lymph nodes

Mucosal: mucosa associated lymphoid tissue (MALT) and mammary glands

1.Spleen:

There are no Afferent lymphatic vessels, which removes bloodstream antigens.

Structure :

Red pulp is the zone of the senescence (aging) in RBCs

Marginal zone: divides the two pulps. It is home to APC Macrophages, APC, and the LB

White pulp: arranged around a central arteriole, with the T-dependent as well as B-dependent zones.

2.Lymphatic nodes:

Lymphatic circulation occurs limited to one direction Tissue Ganglia and Blood.

Structure:

Subcapsular Peripheral (cortical) is rich in LB that is arranged in crowns to make primary follicles, which then change into secondary follicles following an antigenic stimulus

Para-cortical: Thymo-dependent, abundant in LT (between the subcapsular and the medula)

Medullary: mixed zone comprising : LB, LT, macrophages, and plasmocytes.

3.Mucosal related lymphoid tissues (MALT):

Guards against the mucous membranes (respiratory and digestive), urogenital Ocular, etc.).

Tissue of diffuse lymphoid and +/- personalized structures (pay plates Appendix, tonsils ...).

Locally evokes the response of humor that is secretory IgA.

II.CELLS OF SPECIFIC IMMUNITY

T lymphocytes

MATURATION AND DIFFERENTIATION OF LT:

The lymphoid precursor of the bone Marrow into the thymus differentiation and maturation from the medullary cortex.

Trois principales phases:

Double-negative: no CD4, no CD8.

Double positive: CD4 plus CD8:

The thymus cells comprise 85% of the cells

Rearrangement in the genes that encode the chain in the TCR

A TCR of low density is described

Simple positive: the loss either of CD4 or

- Increased TCR/CD3.

Negative selection: removal of thymocytes with TCR detects with very high affinity self peptides.

B. INTRA-THYMIC SELECTION:

Positive selection

It involves TCR (a and B) DP thymocytes and cortical TECs which are expressing MHC I as well as II

Based on the affinity between TCR and MHC. Based on affinity between TCR

Low or high affinity death by apoptosis or deletion.

The cells saved are simply positive CD4 or CD8 and continue their maturation, and they will also pass the negative choice.

2.Negative selection

The medullary part of the corticomedullary junction the presence of antigen-presenting cells and TEC from the medullary

Thymocytes that produce self-peptides and are destroyed by the process of apoptosis, or deletion of clonal cells.

Thymocytes (now maturing LT) quit the thymus and head to Lymphoid Organs II (T-dependent zones) These LT still and waiting to make contact with Ag. Ag are referred to as Naive LT.

C. ACTIVATION OF T-CELLS

The interaction between T-APC and T-APC involves:

1st activation signal 1st activation signal: binding between TCR/CD3 MHC-PP, on one hand, and CD4/CD8 as well as MHC II/MHC I to the contrary.

Second activation signal 2-nd activation signal linkage CD28 - CD86 Leader

The contact with the T-APC triggers activation of enzymes Protein Tyrosine Kinases (PTK) in the contact areas of

Intracytoplasmic regions of TCR/CD3 are with a high concentration of activation motifs that are which are based upon the phosphorylation the Tyrosine

D. LT activation phenotype:

CD25, Alpha chain for the IL-2 receptor

MHC II molecules

CD40L

CTLA4/ CD152

CD71 receptor for transferrin

CD49 is a VLA1 chain, which acts as the laminin receptor

E. LT sub-populations:

LT TCR (beta, alpha)or CD3

LT CD4+ and LT CD8+

CD4 LTs are subdivided in:

Conventional CD4 LTS are express CD25 only upon activation.

CD4 regulators: LT CD4 regulators: release CD25 and CTLA4 in a consistent manner they suppress all immune responses to self-antigens. They also assist to prevent the development of autoimmune diseases and exert their influence by releasing IL10 and TGF beta.

2. LT TCR (gama, delta) :

CD4- and CD8-

They express inhibitory and activated killer receptors similar to NK cells (NKR)

They are also known as the effectors of LT and cytotoxic. They are intraepithelial lymphocytes, IEL.

is a key component in the mucosal immune system.

II. B Lymphocytes

A. Ontogenesis of B cells:

1.) From stem cells to mature LB (non-ag depended lymphopoiesis):

Localization: yolk sac MO, fetal liver the spleen

The molecular mechanism is a rearrangement the Immunoglobulin gene

In the case of MO, maturation takes place through contact with non-lymphoid cells via :

Cell-cell contact via adhesion molecules such as VCAM1 of VLA4 of stromal cells from preLBs

Molecular contact thanks to the development factors CSF+ IL3/IL7

Negative selection: LBs that are not yet that react with self-molecules are eliminated

4 steps : Early pro B, late pro B, pre B, immature B

- Stage: Pro B

BCR Ig genes have not been altered (germline configuration)

- Markers: - CD19 - CD79a = Iga, CD79b = Igb

- Stage: Pre B

BCR: Synthesis, as well as expression m heavy chain IgM by rearranging genes

1.) PreB1 Intracytoplasmic Heavy Chain.

2.) PreB2 Heavy chain expressed on the surface, in very small amounts and pseudo-light chain (substitution)

The pre BCR comprised of two domains: variable: pre B and constant 5.

C. Stade: B immature

BCR: IgM of the complete Surface = BCR

The spleen is located:

immature LBs have the surface IgD mature LBs functionally naive LBs that express IgM and IgD

the entire mass of LBs are renewed each three days (half-life equals 3 days) Except for LBs that are activated by Ag stay alive, and then move into the OL II and pass to the Lymphoid Organs II. They then populate the underlying LB zones, which form the primary Follicles.

2.) from maturing LB and activated LB (Ag dependent lymphopoiesis):

Secondary Locations: secondary LOs

Mechanisms: Somatic Hypermutation as well as isotypic switch and affinity maturation

Course The course is activated. LBs change to primary follicles. Secondary hair follicles

Secondary follicles: made up of

1) Cenrate part = germinal center

Light area: tiny cells, also known as centrocytes.

Dark zone: big cells - centroblasts.

2.) Peripheral portion of the body: mature LB+Follicular Dendritic Cells (FDC) TCD4+ as well as certain macrophages.

LBA activation: Recognition of Ag native Ag with no the presentation (unlike the LT)

1. Thymo-independent activation doesn't require TH2 in order to generate AC (IgM+) and doesn't trigger memory

Type 1: polyclonal proliferative LBs (activation of the receptors that are common for all LBs other than BCR) via mitogenic Ag

Type 2: monoclonal proliferative LBs (BCR activation) with the help of repetitive sugar the determinants

2- Thymo-dependent stimulation : (majority of responses)

The Ag is specifically recognized as Ag through the BCR and internalization

LT-LB cooperation:

- Primary signal: MHC peptide-TCR interaction

Costimulatory signal: B7 - CD28 as well as CD40-CD40L (CD154)

- Cytokine production: IL-4

Effects of this activation

1.) Clonal proliferative

2.) Hypermutation of the somatic tissue :

The enzyme is expressed exclusively within germinal centers. It is which is the cause of these somatic hypermutations.

Centroblasts: changes to the genes that make up the different areas of BCR are not able to have the ability to produce BCR

-Centrocytes are no longer able to be able to deviate or re-express BCR

that have a distinct affinity for that of Ag in comparison to the first

3.) Positive choice: BCR with a the highest affinity to Ag will be able to are able to receive the survival signal

4.) The differentiation of LB into: Plasmocytes + memory LB

5.) Ig class switching: AID is essential for this switch.

Mature LB + AG; activated LB and lymphoblasts as well as memory cells. LB.

B. Genetics of the Antibody reaction:

1. Primary response: First management of Ag

- Latency phase (0-7 days): no antibody production

Increase in the amount of IgM beginning at 7 days

- Plateau phase (D14) Maximum IgM synthesis

A decrease in IgM Synthesis.

In the case of high doses Ag we'll use an IgM

D7 production and IgG production from D7 and IgG.

2. Second response

- The time of latency (1-3 days) is reduced

The plateau can last longer and shrinks slower.

Chapter 15: Cells Of Innate Immunity

MONOCYTE-MACROPHAGE :

03 compartments:

- Medullary: precursors

- Blood: Monocytes

Tissue is the home of macrophages.

Macrophages are derived from blood monocytes. They constitute 8percent of blood leukocytes. 1/2 life time: 12 - 100 hours.

- Lungs, serous membranes: Macrophages

- Liver: Kupffer cell

- Bone: Osteoclast

- CNS: Microglial cell

- Kidney: Mesangial cell

A- Surface markers:

- MHC I and II, CD14+.

Receptors: R-Cytokines R- - Fc IgG (FCγRI, FCγRII) and IgE C3b,C4b receptor (CR1)

LFA-1 - adhesion molecules ICAM-1, LFA-1

B-Molecules that are created :

- Proteolytic enzymes, Elastase, collagenase, and protease

Components of Complement, growth factors, and coagulation factors

- Cytokines (IL-1, IL-6, TNF)

Chemotactic factors, Arachidonic acid's metabolites Oxygen radicals.

c-Function :

1) Phagocytosis (lysosomes +++)

2.) The presentation of the antigen LT

3.) ADCC, an antibody dependent cellular cytotoxicity is a method of encouraging phagocytosis through the RFc Ig

Phagocytosis steps :

pseudopods > phogosomes > phagolysosome
• microorganisms destroyed by

the enzymes and cellular debris that are released via exocytosis.

Antigen presentation:

Peptides resulting generated by Ag degradation are delivered in LTs through MHC molecules

-- IFNy triggers macrophages and increases levels of HLA I II and I molecules. It also increases the production of cytokine by macrophages.

II. POLYNUCLEARS :

The cytoplasm of the polylobed nucleus has granulations that have different affinity to dyes (MGG stain)

Comprised of three types:

A. The neutrophilic polynuclear cell. 60 % to 70% in blood cells.

A phagocytic cell that is short-lived between 4 and 10 hours

- Nucleus segmented, abundant and the cytoplasm is basophilic.

- Enzymes: Myeloperoxidase, collagenase, elastase, lysozyme + oxygen radicals

- The capability to migrate upon receiving the chemotactic signals: 1. phagocytic cells to move

- Phomacocytes are bound and were opsonized with antibodies and complement.

Membrane receptors: R Cytokine (IL-8) and the Rfragment fc of IgG (FcyII and RFCcyIII) and the R-fraction of complement (C3b as well as C5a) (MHC I

Roles: Bactericides of extracellular bacterial species, clearing of immune complexes

B. The eosinophilic Polynuclear Cell 3% leukocytes

Cells that are cytotoxic, located mostly in the tissues (skin muq) as well as in blood circulation that is brief.

Principal agent in battle against specific parasites.

• Participates in anaphylactic reaction and more prevalent in vasculitides with certain.

C. Polynuclear basophils:

Mature cells after exiting the bone marrow.

Expresses receptors for IgE.

A key role in the defense mechanisms against parasites.

IgE-dependent as well as IgE-independent reactions.

III. DENDRITIC CELLS :

Professional Antigen-Presenting Cells are they are the sole ones capable of stimulating an naive LT as well as stimulate memory and naive LB

Ontogeny is a common precursor (CD34+) within MO through two pathways

Myeloid precursors DC1 = interstitial DC

Precursor to lymphoid cells: Plasma cell and lymphoid DC = DC2.

Dendritic cell distribution:

- Blood: Circulating DC

Epithelium Langerhans cell

The Lymphatic Circulation (afferent channels) Cells that are veiled: T-zones of the LOII

- Lymphoid organs (interdigitated cells):

Thymus : Corticormedullary Junction++, a role in the negativity selection in LT

Spleen : periarteriolar sleeves of the white pulp

Lymph nodes paracortex and MALT = subepithelial as well as interfollicular zone

Follicles lymphoid Follicles : (follicular DC) collect immune complexes and expose them to LBs

Surface molecules:

Receptors to capture antigenic toxins TLR and FcyR (CD32 CD32)

- Antigen processing molecules: cathepsin + DC-Lamp

- Antigen presentation molecules: MHC I and II, CD1

Costimulation and adhesion: CD50 and 54 ICAM-1.3,3 CD58 LFA-3 CD80, the CD86 B7-1, 2 and

- Migration: CD 11(abc)+ CD49(d,e cadherins) CCR 1,5,6,7 +CXCR4

Dendritic cell functions:

DCs are found in two different states:

1.) Immature DCs in tissues: not MHCII or function in endocytosis, and the retrieval of antigen

2.) Mature DCs within LOII T-zones: MHCCII display of MHC-Peptide complexes LTs

The steps that dendritic cells take for presenting the antigen those cells with a specific immune system:

1.) Uptake of antigens by a range of methods: endocytosis, macropinocytosis and phagocytosis.

2.) Dendritic cells migrate to lymphoid organs secondary

3.) Priming is the process of reducing Ag protein Ag protein into peptides that are antigenic, and then the association of all of these antigenic peptides to a

The peptides form make up an MHC molecules.

4.) The maturation of dendritic cells

5.) 5. Presentation of Ag into the LT Two pathways: Endogenous Ag (HLA1 and LTCD8) and Exogenous AG (HLA 2-LTCD4)

Immature DC can be found located in the peripheral tissues. It is a is a phagocyte (endocyte) however it is not there, mature DC is located in the II LO. It is in II LO, but is not phagocytic.

The Immature DC is devoid of MHCII surface. After activation, it will come into contact with

-- Langerhans cells exit the epidermis, they join lymph circulation = cells that are veiled after they move with Antigen to the paracortex of lymph nodes and change into interdigitated cells

IV. NATURAL KILLER LYMPHOCYTES :

3rd lymphocyte population non-T, not-B

10 to 15 percent of lymphocytes present in the circulating blood

There isn't a specific receptor to the antigen. cytotoxic action can be directly exhibited without any specificity,

Prior to sensitization, it is not necessary by an Ag

Morphologically: Large granular Lymphocytes: Large size big cytoplasm, intracytoplasmic cytotoxic Granules: Perforin, granzymes

Phenotype: CD56 (adhesion molecule) and CD16a (unlike macrophage CD16b)

Function:

Natural cytotoxicity: antiviral and anti-tumor

Cytotoxicity does not have to be limited to MHC I

Ac-dependent Cytotoxicity

IFNy secretion (macrophage stimulation) and TNFalpha (inflammation)

Receptors :

The inhibitory NK receptors: possessing as their ligand MHC I molecules that are produced by all nucleated healthy cells within the human body.

Active NK receptors: liganded"activating ligand "activating ligand" present on the body's surface cells

Natural cell cytotoxicity receptors (NCR) The NKp30+44+46 receptors are Viral Ligands

Mechanism of action NK:

Two ways to do it:

1) By an activation-inhibition reaction "missing self"

The NK cell acts as an NK cell that is a killer towards

All cells are affected, however they are blocked by the presence of MHC-I

Infected cells, tumor cells as well as viruses are not expressing MHC I. Therefore the inhibitory effect of NK cells is likely to be removed

2.) 2. ADCC (antibody dependent cell toxicity):

- The NK is home to an RFc receptor (RFc = CD16) that recognizes essential fragments that make up IgG

Chapter 16: To Trigger An Immune Response Immunogenicity

It is recognized with an antigen or lymphocyte (T or B) (antigenicity)

Induction of an immune response via the injection of a substance that induces immunity

Antigenic determinant = epitope: site responsible for antigenic reactivity. Antigens generally have many epitopes. A similar structure to paratope (on Antibody)

Hapten:

Molecular weight low, immunegenic, but not antigenic. isolating antigenic factor.

It could become a cause of infection if it is coupled with a huge transport molecules.

Binds to macrophages, LB, and macrophages however, not to LT.

Therefore, all antigens are immunogens However, certain antigens aren't immunogens.

II. CLASSIFICATION OF ANTIGENS :

Origin From: Artificial, Natural (modification of natural

antigens) or Synthetic.

The structure of the substance Particulate or Soluble

Based on the type of the immune reaction produced:

Thymo-dependent antigens:

Of soluble protein nature

humoral response: IgG: high affinity, memory cells

Thymo-independent antigens

type 1: lipopolyprotein

Type 2: Soluble Polysaccharide

Humoral response IgM with low affinity and no memory cells.

III. CONDITIONS OF IMMUNOGENICITY :

A. Antigen-related characteristics :

1. Distance in phylogenetics is the greater distance that the material is to self, the higher its immunegenicity rises

2. Chemical nature

• Inorganic compounds cannot affect lymphocytes.

Organic compound:

- Proteins: most potent immunogens (polymorphism++).

Polyosides and polysaccharides moderately

immunogenic.

Lipids isolated as pur DNA, are They are not immunogenic. They are the haptens.

3. Size and weight of molecules The higher the molecular weight, stronger the immunegenicity.

4. Complexity of the chemical structure: The more complicated an molecule in its

structure, the more prone to immunogenicity it will be.

5. Catabolism: The more slow catabolism, the greater the stimulation of the antigen and the more the immunegenicity grows.

B. The conditions of administration of antigens :

1. Introduction: the best routes for immunization are IM or intradermal, subcutaneous and.

2. Antigen dosage used

Quantity too low = No reaction

A threshold, the reaction is proportional to the volume

Quantity too large > tolerance to infection.

*Repeated administration is needed for a powerful response (principle for booster shots).

3. The use of adjuvants

Improve immunogenicity through the formation of deposit from the antigen which releases slowly. This means that the interaction of the antigen to the active cells will be prolonged.

C. Host-related factors:

The genotype of the recipient: MHC +++: well-responders as well as poor responders.

The development of age-related immune system

Epitopes with a linear structure (sequential) (also known as a conformational epitope):

The epitope of a linear type is detected by the antibody that is on the denatured and native molecule.

The identification of an epitope conformational is lost following the denaturation of a molecule

V.COMPLEMENT SYSTEM

Definition:

Plasma and membrane proteins, thermolabile, with opsonization-phagocytosis activity. Half-life: 24-48hrs. Split into:

Effector proteins

Regulatory proteins

Receptors of the membrane for supplement fractions.

Factor D is circulated in an active condition (intrinsic enzyme activation)

II- Biosynthesis :

Liver : C3, C6, C8, C9, C1inh

Monocytes-Macrophages: C1 to C9, C1inh, B, D, I, H, P

Cells from epithelial tissues: C1

Fibroblasts : C3, C4

III- Nomenclature

Capital letter C, followed by a number e.g. C1 and C2, for the majority of them.

Factor" Factor D: factor B

Once a protein has been cleaved into fragments, they are identified in lower case letters as C2a and C2b.

The tiny fragment is designated with "a" and the big one is marked by "b", the opposite is true for C2.

C1s for C1s. C1r, and C1q are not fragments of degradation however they are subunits.

IV-Experimentation: Whole blood dry tube

Hemolytic activity of 50 (CH50) (CH50) examines the common and classical routes

C3 and C4 assays (they are administered if they are the first to decline) assays: using the method of immunonephelometry

The AP50 test is an alternative pathway 50: The hemolytic test identifies an alternative route (B D and Proberdine)

Assay for Complement Protein: Radial infrared, immunonephelometry, or ELISA

Individual study of various proteins

the classical path

CH50 : 80 to 120 %U/ml

C1inh : 170 to 570 mg/L

C1q : 110 to 200 mg/L

C4 : 150 to 450 mg/L

Track alternative

C3c: 800 to 1800 mg/L

B : 90 to 320 mg/L

V-Activation pathways

1.Classical pathway of complement

Actions of the pathway

Immune complexes++ that's Antibody is IgM or IgG (G1 G2 or G3)

A few Gram-negative bacteria (LipoPolySaccharide) as well as some DNA viruses

CRP, C-reactive protein

Urate crystals and apoptic bodies

Activation proteins:

C1, C2, C4

Regulatory proteins:

C1 inh: separation of C1 through binding C1s and C1r : Tetramer C1inh, C1r, and C1s

C4bp: is able to dissociate C3 convertase via linking to C4b. Cofactor of I

2.Lectin pathway:

Process activators

Indirectly by microorganisms with either N-acetylglucosamine, or terminal mannose residues

Activation proteins:

MBL=C1q / MASP 1 = C1r / MASP 2 = C1s

Regulatory proteins:

C1 inh: dissociation from C1 through binding to C1s and C1r: Tetramer C1inh, C1r, and C1s

C4bp dissociates C3 convertase via linking to C4b. Cofactor of I

3. Alternative route:

Activators of the pathway

Do not require antibodies

Aggregated IgA

Contact with germs directly

Cells infected with viruses

Xenogeneic RBCs

Activation proteins:

C3, B, D,

P (Properdine) : stabilizes C3 convertase

Regulatory proteins:

Factor H and Factor I to limit the spontaneous activation of $C3H_2O$

4. Membrane attack complex: common pathway:

Activation proteins:

C5 C6 C7 C8 C9

Regulatory proteins:

Protein S (vitronectin)

Clusetrin, HRF (CD59)

VI. Complement Activation:

1- The traditional path:

C1 activation:

C1 is circulated in bloodstream in the form of pentamer (C1r-C1s)2 + C1q.

C1q:

Bouquet design of six petals: six heads at each activator location for binding.

Every activator of the classical pathway are identified by C1q.

C1s : a functional unit for C1.

C1r: Serine protease.

It is believed that the presence of 2 IgGs are required to ensure C1 activation. In contrast, only one IgM suffices.

C4 Activation:

The activation of C1s breaks down C4 and releases 2 fragments 2 fragments: C4a (anaphylatoxin) released, and C4b is bound to the activater surface.

C2 Activation:

The C4b that is attached to the activator transforms into a C2 acceptor, i.e. C4b-C2 complex. The C2 that is bound is then the C1's target that cleaves it to : C2b, which can be released; and C2a that remains linked to C4b. Both carry an enzymatic function (serine protease).

The C4bC2a complex is a C3 convertase from the classic pathway

C3 Activation :

C3 convertase breaks down C3 and then releases C3a (anaphylatoxin) that is released as well as C3b that binds C3 convertase.

The C4bC2aC3b Complex = C5 convertase from the classic pathway

C5 C6 C7 Activation

The C5 convertase breaks down C5 and releases C5a anaphylatoxin that releases and C5b which is bound to activater.

C5b interacting with C6 = C5b-C6 that will interact with C7 = trimer C5b C6-C7.

The development of this complex is that proteins turn hydrophobic, which means they may bind to membrane liquids

C7 C8 C9 Activation

The C5bC6-C7 protein that is attached to membrane lipids binds C8 The C5b-C6-C7 complex acts as an C9 receptor. C9.

Many molecules of C9 (6 through 12) become entangled with the membrane attack complex

Membrane C5b-C6C6-C7C8-9n : MAC that is inserted into the bilayer of lipids and is a transmembrane channel which is involved in cell lysis through hyperosmosis.

2. Alternative pathway:

When the liquid phase is present, and in the absence any activity or activation, the C3 molecules are hydrolyzed spontaneously. C3H2O and is akin to C3b (C3b-like).

C3H2O connects with the activator and binds to factor B that will then be divided into two parts ba and bb through the factor D.

The Ba fragments are released in the medium. the Bb and C3H2O are combined to form convertase. It is a different initiation process for the C3 (C3H2OBb)

C3 convertase cuts other C3s into C3a+C3b

C3 attaches to cell's surface and form a the new, solid C3 convertase

(C3bBb) = amplification loop

C3b is bound to C3b-Bb in order and forms the second C5 convertase (C3b)nBb

C5 convertase is able to cleaves C5 to C5a and C5b at that point, the cascade continues to repeat itself

3- Lectins pathway:

Interactions of MBL (mannan bound and lectin) in conjunction with mannose residues N-acetylglucosamines

MBL is related to two components: MASP 1 and MASP 2.

The activation of MBL/MASP, which leads to the development of the classic C3 convertase C4b2a, and it is activated in a manner similar as that of the classic pathway.

VII. The regulation of the system that complements it:

The regulatory proteins block activation and help protect healthy tissues.

They dissociate C3 as well as C5 convertases or breakdown C3b, C4b into inactive fragments C3bi, C3dg, C3d and C4bi

Beyond the regulator proteins, there are also membrane inhibitors.

DAF dissociates C3 from C5 convertases.

CD59 blocks MAC assembly.

MCP CD35 (CR1) is a cofactor in factor I.

VIII. Complement receptors

CR1 (CD35):

Binds to C3b+C4b +

The expression is expressed on: Red blood cells (Mac, PN), Pholocytic (Mac, the PN) L, LT,

The role of this is to clear the circulating ICs

Chapter 17: Behcet's Disease- Painful Mouth And Generic Ulcers

CD55 (DAF) and CD59 (protectin)

Paroxysmal hemoglobinuria nocturnal with RBCs lacking in CD55 and CD59 Lies.

2.) Infections acquired by the body more frequently, caused through exaggerated consumption of supplement proteins

Dessiminated Lupus Erythematosus Auto antibodies

Hepatic insufficiency causes cirrhosis.

Gram-negative sepsis: strong complement activation

Cryoglobulinemia: hypocomplementemia resulting from an activation of the classical pathway

Glomerulonephritis type II is characterized by autoantibodies (nephritic factors) focused against C3 in the alternative pathway

Lipodystrophy partial.

The best method to determine the source of the deficit:

CH50 C3, and C4 normal: cease the investigations.

CH50 C3, and C4 high C4 high: Inflammation and infections

C4, C3 and CH50 diminished

The hyperactivation of the traditional or path of lectin

Insufficiency hepatocellular insufficiency

Two unlikely" genetic deficiencies C1q has been investigated as a possible hereditary cause.

CH50 reduced, C3 decreased C4 normal

activation of the alternative route (catabolize C3 but not through C4)

CH50 decreased, normal C3 increased, C4 decreased

Initiation of the classical pathway

Deficit in C4

Inhibition of C1 (hyperactivity of C1s and therefore an increase in the catabolism of C4)

CH50 reduced, C3 and C4 are normal

Specific deficit in : C1 and C2,

If there is a meningococcal infection in the case of C5 C6 C7 insufficient (C9 deficiency may be the cause of symptoms).

VI.CYTOKINES AND CHEMOKINES:

Cytokines

Cytokine is a signaling molecule

Chemokine is a chemotactic cytokine

Lymphokines : created by LT

Monokines, produced only by macrophages and moncytes

Interleukin is a messenger that helps communicate between immune cell subpopulations

1. General properties:

Low molecular weight, soluble glycoproteins

Antigen-specific non-specific mediators

Short secretion usually at small distances

Pleiotropism The same cytokine could be present in multiple cellular or tissue impacts points

Redundancy: Different cytokines could be able to perform identical functions

Method of action: Autocrine, Paracrine, Endocrine.

2- Receptors:

Receptor-Cytokine binding is much more specific than AC-AG and Rc-Hormone binding.

Structure:

Extracellular domain: conserved

Transmembrane domain: hydrophobic, two to

Three chains:

A-chain: affinity, specificity and

B-chain (possibly g-chain) Signal transduction that is common to a variety of receptors

In the intracellular domain, it is often not with any tyrosine-kinase activities

Type 1:

Hematopoietin receptors

Extracellular domain: 04 cysteines as well as the WSXWS motif

Type 2:

Receptors for interferons

04 cysteines are conserved in the extracellular regions of their domains.

Type 3:

TNF receptors

Different quantity of extracellular domains abundant and homologous to cysteines

Type 4:

Ig Superfamily receptors

immunoglobulin-like domains. Two subgroups
:

The IL1R gene is not involved in tyrosine
protein kinase function

Growth factors: Tyrosine Kinase activation

Type 5:

Chemokines receptors:

07 transmembrane region and G proteins.

3. Transduction pathways for signal
transduction:

The majority of the cytokine receptors have
no an intrinsic tyrosine kinase function and
therefore they are able to recruit intracellular
tyrosines such as Src, and JAK (Janus Kinase)

JAK STAT pathway the main pathways for
transduction used for Receptor Types I and II

The signal transduction chains that are
common among different receptors for

cytokine explain the redundancy of cytokine reactions This issue can be fatal the event of a deficit in IL2Rg:

ILRg deficiency: a severe immune defect that can be fatal the SCID: severe combination immune deficiency

4. Cellular sources of cytokines

The main source of Cytokines

The TH0 test results in: (IL12 INFg) Th1: cell immune system (hypersensitivity IV) and macrophage activation. TNFa.

-- (IL4 10, 10) T2 The TH2 is IL4, 5,6,10 and 13. immune (hypersensitivity I) and LB proliferative

- (IL6, TGFb), TH17: IL17, IL21,22,23, INFg.

- (TGFb) Treg: tolerance.

5. Functional classification:

The Cytokines of Inborn Immunity:

a. Pro-inflammatory:

IL1:

Source: Monocyte-Macrophages, dendritic cells.

Functions:

Liver: Synthesis of acutely inflammatory proteins

Procoagulant activity is increased in the endothelium and adhesion of leukocytes to endothelial cells

OS Resorption, Osteoclast activation Hematopoiesis, osteoclast activation

Pyrogenic and anorexic.

It activates LT, LB and macrophages by cytokine synthesis

The stimulation of the IL-2 receptor and IL-2 secretion

Reduces LPL activity in the adipose tissue

The production of corticosteroids is increased through the adrenal glands.

IL6:

Source: Monocyte-Macrophages, dendritic cells, TH2, endothelial cell.

Functions:

The same action is exhibited in liver endothelium the bone tissue, and bone the marrow. It is also pyrogenic

LBL: differentiation into plasma cells, and maturation of plasma cells Ig Synthesis

TNFa:

Source: Monocyte-Macrophages, dendritic cells, endothelial cell.

Functions:

The first cytokine to be released during inflammatory process

The increase in adhesion molecules that are found on the endothelial cell

The cytotoxic capacity that is present in NK, LTC and macrophage

Proapoptic, moderate antiviral active against parasites and tumors.

b. Antiviral:

IFNa:

Source: Monocyte-Macrophages, LB.

IFNb:

Source: endothelial cell and the fibroblast

Functions: Same for A and B.

Anti-viral and anti-tumor activities

Expression of MHC I increases

It increases the cytotoxic capacity that is present in CLT and NK

The treatment of some illnesses: hepatitis, Kaposi's Sarcoma

B. Cytokines in the immune specific response

IL2:

Source: TH1

Functions:

Growth factor LT

the proliferation of LT4 and LB +, but they are not implicated in the TH1/TH2 polarization

The differentiation of pre-CTLs to CTLs which enhances NK CTL activity.

It is important to note that IL2 has a lot of biological roles with IL15

IFN G:

Source: TH1

Functions:

Divergence of LTH0 to LTH1 through inhibition of the T2 pathway.

Activates: Macrophage, NK and CLT.

The increase in Expression MHC II molecules. MHC II molecules

It has a weak antiviral action.

IL4:

Source: TH2, LB mast cells, and basophils

Functions:

synergy   IL13   synergy   with   IL13: transformation of TH0 to TH2 as well as inhibition of pathways to TH1

LBL: Proliferation, Expression of MHC II and CD23

The key to the switch the switch from IgM > The HSI

IL5:

Source: Th2, mast cells and basophils

Functions:

Synergy between IL4 and IL4: IgE production

The production, the proliferation and activation of activated LBs and transformation in IgA plasma cells.

Eosinophils are eosinophils that grow

IL12:

Source: Dendritic cells, monocytes, macrophages

Functions:

Synergy IFNg and differentiation from Th0 to Th1 through an inhibition of the Th2 pathway.

Proliferation of Th1 as well as the NK cells and boosts the IFNg synthesizing capacity of these cells.

C. Regulation cytokines C. Regulatory cytokines: Cytokines that are anti-inflammatory

IL10:

Source: Th2, LB, LT, monocytes.

Functions:

In the context of macrophages and Th1, Immunomodulatory and anti-inflammatory cytokine.

Chapter 18: Mif Blocks Macrophage Migration

MCF stimulates monocyte migration

MAF stimulates macrophages

Utilization of cytokines as therapeutic agents

Utilization of cytokines :

- IL-2: metastasized kidney cancer, prostate cancer, AIDS

- - IL-10: Crohn's disease

IFN alpha: hepatitis B and C

-- IFN beta IFN beta: MS

Utilize anti-cytokines :

- Anti- TNF: RA

- Anti- CD25: Organ transplantation

- Anti- IL1 and Anti-IL5: Asthma

II. Chimiokines:

Chemotactic Cykines: Recruitment of leukocytes into the inflammatory sites

Produced by stimulation of TNF, IL-1

Various sources: hepatocytes, fibroblasts, leukocytes, epithelial cells

The most important chemokine is IL-8 . It's also known as alpha-chimiokine , which is synthesized by epithelial cells. its primary function is to facilitate the recruitment to PNN (Pyogen)

Size small (90 to 130 in aa) as well as four cysteine residues that are conserved.

Sorting according to N-terminal residues: 50 distinct chemical chemokines are distributed across 20 diverse receptors

Four distinct families of chemokines with 20 to 45% of homology

CxC: the first two cysteines, separated by an An

CXCL8 (IL-8): Neutrophils

CXCL7 (NAP-2): Basophils

CXCL12 (SDF-1): LB

CC: first two adjacent cysteines:

CCL2 (MCP1) : Monocytes

CCL5 (Rantes) : Monocytes

CCL1 (eotaxine) : Oesinophiles

The cysteine 1 is replaced with another AA

XCL1 and XCL2: Lymphocytes and NK

CXXXC : 3 random AAA within the first two cysteines

CX3C L1 (Fractalkine) is a protein that allows for the adhesion of leukocytes to endothelial cell surfaces.

www.ingramcontent.com/pod-product-compliance
Lightning Source LLC
Chambersburg PA
CBHW062141020426
42335CB00013B/1297